# The Truck & Bus Driver Sleep Apnea Handbook

*What Every OTR Driver Needs To Know About Sleep Apnea*

Bruce Maxim

# The Truck & Bus Driver Sleep Apnea Handbook

## *What Every OTR Driver Needs To Know About Sleep Apnea*

Visit our website at *www.SleepApneaHandbook.com* and leave a review. Please do the same at Amazon as my objective is to help as many drivers as possible by providing information they can easily understand and use, and to encourage them to take the most appropriate action in order to improve their health.

Special discounts on bulk quantities of this and other publications by the author are available to corporations, professional associations, health care organizations and other qualifying groups upon contacting the author by email at *Info@SleepApneaHandbook.com*.

**Disclaimer:** This book is intended strictly to provide information based on the personal experience of the author. It is not intended to formally diagnose or otherwise provide medical or dental advice. As a result of potentially acting upon the information presented in this book, you will have made a personal decision to do so. To accept treatment of any description including surgery should be done so only upon the advice of the treating physician or dentist. The author shall not accept liability or responsibility for any person with respect to loss, injury or damage caused by or alleged to be caused by information contained in this publication.

# Dedication

To those drivers who died on the road while performing their everyday jobs, and to those who were just unlucky victims. This is for those who unfortunately did not have this information in order to benefit from it, and for those who did have it but simply failed to act on it.

# Contents

# Introduction

Every day there are more and more books, medical papers, and articles available on the subject of *Sleep Apnea* than ever before. It is somewhat rare to find one that is not predominantly about *snoring* at the outset, even though they all tend to get around to the underlying issue of sleep disorders. To discover you have a sleep disorder is obviously the much more serious side of what is primarily a social inconvenience. Not to minimize the snoring issue because *it is a red flag* for a potential sleep apnea diagnosis. If you're suffocating and starving for oxygen while trying to sleep you are virtually certain to be snoring loudly. Thankfully, the noise you make while snoring and the inconvenience caused to whomever is within earshot, may just save your life. **Not everyone who snores has sleep apnea, but just about everyone who has sleep apnea snores.**

This book is intended for, but not limited to, those who make their living as professional drivers, and especially those who operate larger commercial vehicles. By extension, you should share this book with your families and friends because no one is exempt. In fact, they too can easily be adversely affected by second hand snoring in much the same way. Think about what you undoubtedly have learned about second hand smoke in recent years.

My focus is to get the attention of those who drive transport trucks and highway buses over long and boring stretches of highway for a mind-numbing number of miles or kilometres, and hours. This information applies equally to commercial airline pilots, city transit drivers, railway engineers, heavy equipment operators, police officers, and shift workers in general. In fact, anyone who drives at all should pay attention and take action if necessary.

The book is also intended for *all* of the transportation companies and organizations that employ you. Most of them currently appreciate the paradigm shift and culture change that relates to sleep apnea that is coming fast, and in many cases has already arrived.

What is *not* new to the transportation industry at large are *Drug and Alcohol Testing* and *Distracted Driving* issues. Those matters are currently of equal importance as *Rules of the Road* and *Seatbelt Laws* in terms of priority, so it follows then that you can **expect mandatory testing** for sleep disorders across the industry.

Truck and bus drivers, pilots and anyone else who operates a commercial vehicle or other heavy equipment for a living will soon discover that, license or not, unless they subject themselves to a sleep study, they will never be a 'new hire' again as it *will* become a condition of employment. When your license comes up for renewal and you have to undergo your usual department of transport-mandated medical, it's a certainty you will be required to undergo a *polysomnogram (PSG)*, or overnight sleep test.

Employers are now much less inclined to be tardy in this evolution. It won't take more than one single lawsuit where an accident investigation reveals a driver had a pre-existing sleep disorder, yet the employer either failed to screen, failed to test, or otherwise turned a blind eye and put that driver on the road in order for that company to become proactive in this regard.

This book is intended for those who rely on their license to hold their job, and who are literally terrified that if they come forward, or if anyone ever finds out that they either might or do have sleep apnea, that they would be at risk of losing that license. They've heard stories of their colleagues who have had their licenses suspended. They know what those same colleagues went through to get reinstated, and they want no part of it so they remain silent. They want no interruption in terms of earning a living as they simply need to maintain their livelihood.

I know of instances where sleep therapy professionals have attended transportation association, union meetings and employee 'lunch and learn' sessions for the purpose of educating drivers on this subject. The reception they get is often as if the 'sleep police' have just arrived to interrogate the drivers. This reaction is strictly out of fear of being discovered, and my goal is to try and help you overcome that fear.

Please read carefully and be assured that you will not lose your license as long as you have been formally assessed and diagnosed, are being properly treated *and* you are compliant with that prescribed treatment.

**This book is intended as a *Call To Action* for all Transportation Workers and the Companies That Employ Them**

# Chapter One

## Sleep Apnea and the Transportation Industry

*I have a diagnosed severe Obstructive Sleep Apnea (OSA).* I am a commercially licensed driver (CDL) and a licensed pilot. I was first formally diagnosed by way of a hospital sleep study at age 46, but based on what I know now I am certain that I was first afflicted by around age 39 (and probably earlier). I have more than 40 years working in transportation including the airlines, airport management, the trucking industry, and the *'Not For Profit'* sector as a transportation executive and expert of sorts.

You will soon come to know if you are a candidate for OSA and my goal is simply to convince you to get tested. I will also demystify the subject of sleep apnea and try to isolate it (at least somewhat) from the issue of snoring as a stand-alone problem.

I place much more importance on getting properly diagnosed and treated for a potential sleep apnea than simply seeking a remedy for snoring. Your situation might be that your snoring consistently annoys others who are unwilling to continue tolerating the noise you make, so they are pressuring you to have it dealt with. In doing so, as with a rather large number of instances you may discover that you also happen to have sleep apnea. That sleep apnea is often a silent killer.

If you drive a truck or bus for a living, you should know that the number of both fatal and non-fatal accidents in this group is skyrocketing. Many accidents and deaths fail to get properly blamed on a driver's sleep apnea because it is inherently difficult to prove after the fact if the driver has not previously been diagnosed.

As an analogy, imagine a physical assault where a person is stabbed by way of a large icicle that dangled then fell from an eaves trough. The police investigate but fail to locate or identify the weapon used. The truth is they may never figure out what the weapon was that was used, or what really happened!

The larger issue of sleep apnea resides right across the transportation industry. For example, flying a commercial jet for a 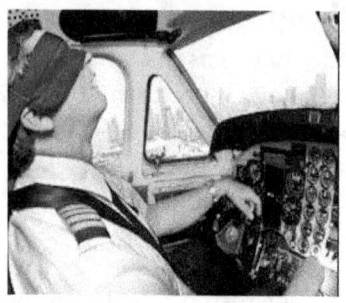 living sounds sexy, but when there are no mechanical issues to deal with, no weather concerns to speak of, no alerts going off once on autopilot and at cruising altitude, it *can* be a much less exciting occupation than you would think. Both transcontinental and longer haul intercontinental flights can get pretty boring after take-off and climb out until just before the decent and landing phases. The only advantage is that there is more than one pilot, plus there is a cabin crew to provide human interaction and distractions while on route to the destination. You might be moving along at over 500 MPH, but you can't tell. It can be as routine as driving a commercial vehicle if it's your everyday job.

The railway industry is not exempt. The next time you ride a commuter train where the locomotive is pushing you from behind, try to sit in the front car looking out the forward window at the seemingly endless and hypnotizing tracks you are traveling on. Or try the same thing underground in the leading car of a subway train. Pretend it's your everyday job and try to project how it would affect you if you experience daytime drowsiness as a rule. There are numerous examples like this for all of the aforementioned work groups.

*I want to tell you my own story about going through this process,* mostly because in the beginning I had no idea how serious OSA was. I know that for those who are yet to be diagnosed, the majority simply don't realize the health risk they are taking. There are a few other reasons too.

Several years ago a friend of mine with a family that included a couple of young children, held down two jobs to make ends meet. His second job was playing guitar in a bar band, usually weekends plus two or three nights through the week. As you can imagine, on the nights he played at a club he would generally finish up just before 1:00 AM and then drive home to grab a few hours sleep before heading off to his day job.

This particular night he was driving home along the expressway minding his own business when the traffic slowed down for some overnight construction work up ahead. When he was almost slowed down to a crawl, an 18-wheeler drove right into the back of him at about 60 MPH. Long story short, the police report concluded that the driver fell asleep at the wheel on the basis that there was no mechanical fault found with the rig, and other witnesses said there was no attempt at braking. Two fatalities in one event!

Secondly, I would need an accountant to calculate how many times I have been personally startled to full alertness each time the tires on my car came into contact with the rumble strips along the side of the highway. At one time or another everyone has encountered this warning device when drifting onto the shoulder area. Even though I have been successfully treated for my sleep apnea, on long commutes I sometimes still tire easily. I learned my lesson a long time ago. Today, at first nod I stop for a fifteen minute powernap - no exceptions.

My biggest incentive for sharing this information, and to put it into perspective, is that the study of sleep disorders and sleep apnea in particular is still in its infancy. No one should feel isolated over a lack of subject knowledge because until about five years ago medical schools didn't even teach this information. Go ahead and ask your doctor if I am exaggerating. Most doctors had less than an hour of lecture on the subject, so it is not surprising that public and patient education has been abysmal, to say the least. That's why you have to be proactive and take the initiative to get tested. If you don't, before long your employer will likely do it for you. Would it not be better for you if **you** controlled that process? Besides, why ignore the signs and make yourself sick?

If you already know that it's possible that you *may* have a sleep disorder, what intelligent person would risk killing themselves and possibly doing the same to other innocent people traveling on the same highways by remaining undiagnosed? You are as much as nine times more likely to cause an accident if you have a sleep disorder. And as they like to say on television: "....but wait, there's more!"

Your career in transportation aside, that is only a part of what is at risk. If you never drove another truck, bus, car, boat, plane, bike, or whatever again, this information still applies to you and your health. Untreated sleep apnea is *directly* related to hypertension (high blood pressure), the resulting heart disease, and strokes. There is also a direct correlation to diabetes, bi-polarism, TMD (or TMJ which is temporomandibular jaw joint disorder) along with the resulting headaches, bruxism (grinding of teeth at night), and acid reflux issues (GERD). The most recent correlation is with cancer as it is known to perpetuate abnormally fast tumor growth due to poor sleep quality. Personally, my attention would have been piqued all the way back at heart attack and stroke.

I don't want to bombard you with the inevitable statistics until you can see how you fit into them. As I said, there is not a long history on the study of sleep disorders, so hopefully you will view this information as fairly recent and relevant. I'll discuss causes and connect the underlying snoring issue as I expand on how serious sleep apnea can really be in terms of your overall health and longevity. We will discuss diagnoses (both your own informal diagnosis as well as a proper medical diagnosis) and outline treatment options.

As far as sleep apnea is concerned, there is not really a cure per se, but it is quite treatable. In fact, you will learn that your dentist (or at least some dentists) may be just as valuable in providing a solution as the sleep specialist doctor. If you have a regular dentist, there is a section that you can take to your him/her in order to provide incentive for them to get involved in sleep therapy treatment if currently they are not.

It is becoming widely known that there are not enough sleep specialists to meet the medical demand, and there are not enough dentists who understand their potential role in treating sleep apnea by incorporating snoring and sleep therapy into their existing practice. For a very long time, the medical and dental vocations have not seen eye to eye on the subject of treatment for sleep apnea. It is still an ongoing issue, but alliances are beginning to spawn between the two communities.

If your dentist currently cannot help you, hand him/her the book or mention where you got your copy, then encourage him/her to expand their practice by learning to screen and treat even their existing patients for snoring and sleep issues. Then go and find one in your area that can help you, or contact the author to refer you. The market size has already grown off the map, and it is only going to get bigger. Hopefully this information will get to you just in time.

# Why are Commercial Drivers in a Special Risk Group?

Tell me this has *never* happened to you while driving. Your eyelids droop into a pair of lampshades, your head starts bobbing, you can't stop yawning and your vision begins to blur. You begin to blink at three times the normal rate before you catch yourself leaving the lane you're in and then quickly jerk the steering wheel to straighten out. You just lucked out and recovered, but sooner or later there will be a different outcome.

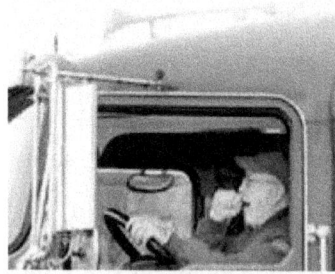

National Sleep Foundation research suggests that 60% of Americans have driven while feeling sleepy and 37% admit to actually having fallen asleep at the wheel in the past year. There is much data available and most reveals that there are virtually no cultural differences amongst the populations of North America, the UK, Europe and Australia when it comes to sleep, obesity, driving in general; and particularly driving to earn a living. The data is consistent, prototypical, and totally applicable to most countries whose economies and travelers are largely reliant on their highways. You can extrapolate data originating in the any of the aforementioned locales and make it accurately reflect wherever you live.

For example, to me there is zero difference between the USA and Canada when it comes to driving. With a North American population of about 460 million (USA 314M, Mexico 112M, Canada 34M) versus 62 million in the UK, those percentages more or less apply. If you want statistics go to *www.truckinginfo.net*, but to summarize there are about 3.5 million truck drivers in the USA and about 250,000 in Canada. About 60% are *Over the Road*

(OTR) or long haul tractor-trailer drivers. In the USA each year there are about 5,000 fatal accidents with trucks involved. The real issue is that truck drivers with sleep issues are a public danger. So are bus drivers (highway and transit), commercial pilots, railway engineers (commuter and long haul) and steamship pilots. If anyone operating a vehicle of any description in any of these groups gets drowsy on the job, they are morally obligated to get diagnosed. If you don't, not only do you put innocent people's lives at risk, but you stupidly risk your own longevity and overall health.

Did you know that various studies of long-haul truck drivers continuously find more than 50% symptomatic of sleep apnea? In fact, one such study going all the way back to 1992 that was reported at the European Sleep Research Society Conference in Helsinki, suggested that the study group of truckers revealed that a whopping 87% of them had at least some sign(s) of sleep apnea. They also said that when a trucker dies in a traffic accident, they take an additional 4.3 other victims to their demise.

Conservatively, of those who actually get tested result in about 30% that are actually diagnosed with sleep apnea. This is not lost on the department of transport approved doctors who perform your mandatory medical every few years. When your license comes up for renewal, you would be prudent to take the wind out of his/her sails by being proactive and doing a preliminary self-diagnosis (described in a later chapter).

Start thinking, do I snore? Am I often sleepy in the daytime? Has anyone told me that I stop breathing while asleep at night? Do I have a body mass index (BMI) greater than 30 that suggests obesity? Is my blood pressure higher than 140/90? Do you really want to wait for your employer or doctor to tell you that your commercial driver's license is on the line? Don't wait to be told, get diagnosed and treated accordingly.

# What are Employers Doing About the Problem?

*Employers fear lawsuits, threats to health and safety, and their bottom lines?* It is estimated that about 15% of the population are chronically ill with various sleep disorders, plus as many as an additional 10% experience intermittent sleep-related problems. Sleep apnea is the cause of most excessive daytime sleepiness experienced by these people. This is largely as a result of demanding work schedules (think shift work) and various other lifestyle factors. Today, industry productivity losses are in the billions of dollars.

Did you know that *Sleep Deprivation* has been found to have contributed to the grounding of the Exxon Valdez, the explosion of the space shuttle Challenger, and the nuclear reactor disasters at both Chernobyl and Three Mile Island? Did you know there are marked increases in human job-related errors during the second half of night shifts that have been documented in studies of gasworks employees, drivers, pilots and train engineers?

*To be clear, not all those who are sleep deprived will be found to have sleep apnea*; but those who have been diagnosed with sleep apnea will consistently be deprived of sleep. There is a difference. When it comes to commercial drivers, all trucking and busing companies are virtually certain to employ drivers with serious but undiagnosed and untreated sleep disorders. They know they have to get it under control or one day be shut down for failure to act given that they already have this knowledge. Don't wait for that to happen, rather be proactive and look after yourself first.

In western world studies, the problems are the same no matter what country you live in. Here are some more interesting facts about the impact of sleep disorders in the transportation industry:

- The NTSB found that nearly one-third of all driver/fatal traffic accidents had sleepiness as their probable cause. The drivers in this sampling had an average of only 5.5 hours of sleep during their preceding sleep periods: 2.5 hours less than the average reported by truckers with non-fatigue related accidents.

- One of every five drivers admits to having fallen asleep at least once behind the wheel.

- One British study found that 16-20% of all police-reported MVAs were sleep-related.

- In a Swedish study (after correcting for miles driven) individuals with full sleep apnea symptoms had twelve times as many accidents.

- A British study showed that 93% of those drivers diagnosed were at fault in one or more accidents among distance truck drivers (and who were recently reported as having the highest on-the-job mortality rate of any profession for the third straight year).

- Those working irregular hours are reported to have twice as many accidents.

- The NTSB cited pilot fatigue as a cause or contributing factor in 69 plane accidents, with 67 deaths between 1983-1986 alone.

- Night shift flight simulator performance has been found to be impaired to a degree comparable to that produced by a blood alcohol level of 0.05%.

- Operator fatigue was a major factor in the near-disastrous attempted launch of the space shuttle Columbia in 1986 (accidental drainage of 18,000 lbs of liquid oxygen escaped detection until only 31 seconds before liftoff). As previously mentioned, just three weeks later the space shuttle Challenger exploded. Launch managers had been seriously sleep-deprived. A Presidential Commission cited ground crew fatigue as a significant factor in cause of that disaster.

- *The skipper of the World Prodigy, which dumped 300,000 barrels of oil into Narragansett Bay, admitted to not having slept for 36 hours. Also previously referred to, the NTSB ultimately determined that a primary cause of the Exxon Valdez disaster was sleepiness on the part of its third mate.*

- *Sleep attacks on the job have been documented via EEG monitoring of night shift workers (including locomotive engineers).*

This could be an endless list. As stated in a Time magazine cover story more than 20 years ago, they said: "Sleepy workers are dangerous, less productive, and a major source of increased healthcare costs and corporate liability. Studies of workplace and transportation industries reveal that human error causes up to 90% of accidents, with inadequate sleep representing a major factor in that human error." We know a lot more about sleep disorders and treatments now than we did then, even though it is still almost out of control.

## Hours of Service Rules versus Hours of Sleep

It doesn't matter what mode of transportation you work in, where you are based, or whether operating a truck, bus, train, or plane. You are subject to 'Hours of Service' Rules. They exist for safety reasons and serve their purpose, but only to a degree. While not irrelevant, they are no replacement for identifying and mitigating a potential sleep disorder.

It is expected that on average, a commercial driver should cover about 600 miles per workday. The math is fairly simple if you account for stops and starts, biological breaks, up-shifting and down-shifting and the rest of the things an OTR driver goes through in a day. If he is allowed to drive for 10 hours at an average of 60 MPH, we get 600 miles daily for purposes of this discussion. I personally know companies, and in particular owner-operators, who will tell you that they would be broke in no time at that rate, but it's easier to tell the story if we just go with those numbers for now.

The business end of your vehicle is your office and the driver's seat is you at your desk. You're not allowed to read a book, surf the net, text or email on your smart phone, or do anything else that is not directly related to driving. You do this for at least 10 hours each day that you work. If you did not have a single symptom of sleep apnea and were the epitome of health, you cannot listen to enough music, news, audio books, or afford to gab on the phone (never mind the cost of doing this) to keep you totally alert, not daydreaming or deep in thought. This is very tiring in and of itself, and that is for a totally fit person.

When a driver eventually does get home, they need to recharge their batteries and they need to catch up on sleep and total relaxation before hitting the road again. For a driver with no apparent sleep disorder, the amount of sleep required to completely recharge your system will vary from person to person. If you have kids, you might know that a baby sleeps for a much as 21 hours a day. Your lazy teenagers sleep for about 10 to 11 hours daily if you let them. For the average adult, this drops down to about 8 hours a day (or slightly less).

If you are deprived of the correct amount of sleep for yourself, it will upset your physiological systems including hormones, immune system, blood pressure regulation, digestive system and waste production. Physiological processes tend to work on a 24 hour cycle. Going to sleep and waking up in the morning signals your biological clock to keep all the above noted processes in sync. If the process is disrupted because of shift work or some sleep disorder, the body will reflect this disturbance. From day to day, the hours of service a truck driver operates by are seldom the same 10 to 12 hours on the clock. This is tantamount to working shifts.

*Shift workers have higher incidents of digestive disorders, headaches and some types of cancer.* They are more prone to everything health negative. Some experts will argue that you need nine hours of sleep consistently to be at your most alert level. I personally do not know a human alive in the transportation workforce that regularly gets that amount of sleep. Notwithstanding, when you superimpose a sleep disorder on top of that, you can see the potential for problems.

When a long-haul commercial driver falls asleep at the wheel and crashes, statistics say that an average of four more people will lose their lives along with him. Driving sleepy therefore, is equivalent to driving drunk – and there *are* laws against driving drunk. How many years do you think it will take before "hours of service" rules will be replaced by some sort of automated device that will not let you start the ignition on your rig without passing some sort of 'sleep breathalyser?' That's probably an exaggeration for now, but I'm not so sure in the future.

*In the matter of Obstructive Sleep Apnea detection*, one of the largest trucking firms in the USA with over 15,000 drivers was one of the first to go down this road. In 2006, Schneider National stepped up efforts to screen and test drivers for sleep apnea. Subject to certain compliance factors, they will fund treatment for their drivers thus eliminating two of the barriers for drivers arbitrarily seeking diagnoses. Those barriers are, the fear of a loss of license *and* the cost of treatment not covered by a health plan. Schneider recognized the fact that without enough healthy drivers, they will have equipment unavoidably parked which will negatively impact the bottom line. Since then, some other notable trucking and bus companies have joined in and adopted the concept.

Driving is a sedentary lifestyle, often with days and weeks away from home, long wait times for loads, a truck-stop diet, obesity, a disproportionate number of smokers, and an aging driver group who become more prone to developing sleep apnea after age 40. This is exacerbated by having fewer new drivers coming along for all sorts of other reasons.

## Why Not Take the Bus?

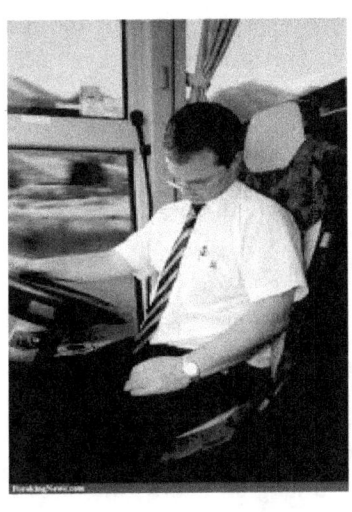

In October of 2012, a tour bus went out of control on Interstate 80 in New Jersey and flipped over (luckily) in a marshy area injuring 23 of 57 on board. No one died and there was no apparent reason for the crash other than driver error. What is happening these days when there is no apparent cause for an accident, investigators tend to conclude that fatigue, or worse, literally falling asleep at the wheel is the primary reason for the accident. The driver in this case said he was cut off, but there was no evidence or witnesses to that effect.

Passengers entering into a lawsuit against the tour operator, bus company (both one and the same), as well as the driver, claim he was either talking or texting on his cell phone, or using his pager. Investigators seem to have ruled that out too.

Looking a little deeper, the Canadian bus company was operating in the USA without a permit because their insurance had lapsed the previous July. It was also discovered that the company had racked up five citations related to fatigued driving, most recently in May of 2012 for 'hours of service' violations. You can see where this is all going. With no clear cause in future accidents, driver fatigue and specifically sleep apnea will be front and centre. As the expression goes: "It's time to smell the coffee if you're the one driving the bus."

Previously in New York City in March of 2011, another tour bus went out of control after drifting off the interstate highway and ended up on its side having sheared off the top of the bus on two signposts, killing 15 and critically injuring eight more of the 31 passengers. The bus company had two previous accidents in each of the two preceding years. During that same time, they too had been cited five times for 'fatigued driving.' No longer are these events viewed as simple log book violations. There *is* a problem and everybody is slowly waking up to that fact.

It's not just tour bus drivers who are being tagged with suspected sleep issues. In Pennsylvania, early in 2012, a school bus driver with 45 kids on board turned left in front of an oncoming car killing a passenger and seriously injuring the driver of the car. Five students also suffered injuries, but there's a kicker as revealed by an onboard camera. The school bus driver had just run 10 stop signs and was totally fatigued after working an overnight shift as a security guard (there's a snooze waiting to happen). It was learned that this driver had caused a previous fatal accident 13 years earlier killing a two year old.

What do you think school bus operators are thinking these days as they try to recruit drivers? Awareness of sleep apnea and other sleep disorders is at or near the top of the list and jobs will be even harder to come by as recruiters look for undiagnosed cases of sleep apnea in potential new hires.

# The '2012 Sleep In America Poll' (National Sleep Foundation)

In addition to truck and bus drivers, now included are pilots, train operators, transit, truck, taxi, and limo drivers. In its 2012 poll, the National Sleep Foundation asked transportation professionals about their work performance and sleep habits. The document is 83 pages long, but here are the highlights:

▫ *About one-fourth of train operators and pilots admit that sleepiness has affected their job performance at least once a week.*

▫ *This is the first poll to ask transportation professionals, including pilots, train operators, and truck, bus, taxi and limo drivers, about their sleep habits and work performance.*

▫ *The study found that pilots and train operators are the most likely to report sleep-related job performance and safety problems.*

▫ *One in five pilots admit that they have made a serious error, and about one in six train operators and truck drivers say that they have had a "near miss," due to sleepiness.*

▫ *The study drew at least one federal-level response: "The results of the NSF poll should serve as a literal 'wake-up call,'" said Deborah Hersman, chairman of the National Transportation Safety Board. "Inadequate sleep puts lives at risk — we see this over and over in our accident investigations. Improving the quantity and quality of sleep can improve safety and ultimately save lives."*

▫ *Managing human fatigue has been on the National Transportation Safety Board's Most Wanted List of transportation safety improvements since the list was created in 1990. As a result of its accident investigations, the agency has issued nearly 200 fatigue-related recommendations to address such areas as hours-of-service requirements, scheduling policies, and diagnosis and treatment of sleep disorders.*

*▫ In the poll results bus drivers were grouped with taxi and limo drivers. School bus drivers accounted for about 43 percent of the respondents in the bus/taxi/limo category. Transit, charter and other types of bus drivers accounted for 35 percent, while taxi and limo drivers were about 22 percent.*

*▫ The bus/taxi/limo group seemed to fare better than others in some key issues. Only 10 percent of them said that sleepiness has affected their job performance at least once a week, compared with 23 percent of pilots, 26 percent of train operators and 15 percent of truck drivers.*

*▫ Seven percent of bus/taxi/limo drivers admit to having made a serious error on the job due to sleepiness, compared with 20 percent of pilots, 9 percent of train operators and 6 percent of truck drivers.*

*▫ Twelve percent of bus/taxi/limo drivers admit to having had a "near miss" at work due to sleepiness.*

For a summary of the poll findings, click here , or if you're reading hard copy go to www.sleepfoundation.org and type 2012 NSF Poll in the search box to see the document.

# Is There a New Role for On-board Cameras?

One final thing to think about in terms of driving for a living and keeping your job when you know you likely have a sleep apnea issue, but are afraid to deal with it. In Washington DC this year, the media has learned that special cameras on Metro buses have caught 68 incidents of drivers briefly nodding off behind the wheel over the course of 19 months.

Half of those drivers who briefly fell asleep were working both morning and afternoon shifts which can add up to a 16-hour day, or what's referred to as a split shift. This is prototypical of most city transit companies. They will tell you that split shifts are necessary to operate the system and drivers have rest time in between their morning and afternoon runs. Split-shifts are a way of life in the city transit industry and are the only way to run an economic service.

In fairness, those 68 incidents represent less than 1 percent of the 370,000 trips a month, but how many accidents need to happen that the public hears about now that they have this revealing information?

No transit company in any city wants bad press, so what do you suspect they might do about it? Appropriately, the 68 drivers involved in these incidents were all sent for medical examinations and for help with sleep management issues before they went back on the road. In future, companies are going to have to be more proactive, so don't wait for that. Get tested on your own.

Just to review, *Sleep Deprivation* is a condition that occurs if you simply do not get enough sleep. *Sleep Deficiency* is a broader concept and occurs not only if you're sleep deprived, but also if you sleep at the wrong time of day, don't get all the types of sleep your body needs, or you have an actual sleep disorder that *prevents* you getting enough sleep and/or causes poor sleep quality.

Sleep Apnea is a common disorder in which you have one or more pauses in breathing or shallow breaths while you sleep. It is usually a chronic (ongoing) condition that *disrupts* your sleep and results in light sleep at best. Sleep apnea often goes undiagnosed as doctors usually cannot detect the condition during routine office visits. Also, there is no blood test that can help diagnose the condition. Most people who have sleep apnea don't know they have it because it only occurs during sleep. A family member or bed partner might be the first to notice signs of sleep apnea. In fact, 'witnessed apneas' theoretically should start a fast track to getting a proper diagnosis if the person with the sleep issue is smart.

# Chapter Two

## A 'Glossary of Terms'

## To Help You Understand the Book

*There are many more medical terms relating to the subject of sleep apnea than you'll ever need to know, but these relate specifically to this material and will assist you with reading and understanding the rest of the book.*

**Adenoids:** Similar to tonsils but located above and behind them.

**AHI:** Apnea/Hypopnea Index is used to assess the severity of sleep apnea based on the total number of complete cessations (apnea) and partial obstructions (hypopnea) of breathing occurring per hour of sleep. These pauses in breathing must last for 10 seconds and are associated with a decrease in oxygenation of the blood. In general, the AHI can be used to classify the severity of disease (mild 5-15, moderate 15-30, and severe greater than 30).

**Airway:** The path that air follows to get into and out of the lungs. The mouth and nose are the normal entry and exit ports for the airway. Entering air then passes through the back of the throat (pharynx) and continues through the voice box (larynx), down the trachea, to finally pass through the bronchi.

**Airway Obstruction:** Partial or complete blockage of the above. Causes include the presence of foreign matter, allergic reactions, infections, anatomical abnormalities, and trauma. If you are not breathing you are considered apneic.

**Apnea:** The absence of breathing (respiration).

**Apnea Event:** Failure to breathe that lasts for more than 10 seconds.

**Apnea Index:** The number of apnea events per hour which is a measure of the severity of the sleep apnea.

**Apnea plus Hypopnea Index:** The total number of apnea and hypopnea events per hour which is also a measure of the severity of the sleep apnea.

**Arrhythmia:** Variation from the normal rhythm of the heartbeat.

**Atherosclerotic:** Pertaining to atherosclerosis, the process of progressive thickening and hardening of the walls of arteries from fat deposits on their inner lining. Atherosclerotic heart disease is the leading cause of death and is frequently related to sleep apnea.

**Bariatric:** Pertaining to the study, prevention, or treatment of being overweight.

**BIPAP:** Same as CPAP but has different pressure setting for exhalation.

**Blood Pressure:** The pressure of blood within the arteries. It is produced primarily by the contraction of the heart muscle. Measurement is recorded by two numbers, first (systolic pressure) measured *after* the heart contracts and is *highest*; second (diastolic pressure) is measured *before* the heart contracts and is *lowest*. Elevated BP is called "hypertension."

**CPAP:** Continuous positive airway pressure, which is considered medically as the gold standard treatment for obstructive sleep apnea.

**CSA:** Central sleep apnea that is caused by some irregularity in the brain's control of breathing.

**Carbon Dioxide:** A gas which is the bi-product of metabolism that collects in tissue, is cleared by blood within the veins, is carried by hemoglobin in the red blood cells, and removed from the body via the lungs in the exhaled air ($CO_2$).

**Cardiac:** Having to do with the heart.

**Congenital:** A condition that is present at birth, whether or not it is inherited.

**Congestive Heart Failure:** Inability of the heart to keep up with the demands placed on it, with failure of the heart to pump blood with normal efficiency. The heart is unable to provide adequate blood flow to other organs, such as the brain, liver, and kidneys.

**Deviated Septum:** Failure of the nasal septum to be in the center of the nose and divide the nasal passages evenly. Deviation of the nasal septum may be congenital (present at birth) or acquired (occur later). It causes an airway obstruction and can be corrected with surgery.

**EDS:** Excessive daytime sleepiness which is a neurological disorder in which there is a sudden recurrent uncontrollable compulsion to sleep.

**Fatigue:** A condition characterized by a lessened capacity for work and reduced efficiency of accomplishment, usually accompanied by a feeling of weariness and tiredness.

**Gastroesophageal Reflux:** The return of stomach contents back up into the esophagus. This frequently causes heartburn because of irritation of the esophagus by stomach acid.

**GERD:** Gastroesophageal reflux disease.

**High Blood Pressure:** A repeatedly elevated blood pressure exceeding 140 over 90 mmHg (also known as hypertension).

**Hypopnea:** Literally, under-breathing or breathing that is shallower or slower than normal. It is distinct from apnea in which there is <u>no</u> breathing.

**Insomnia**: Inadequate or poor-quality sleep due to difficulty falling asleep, waking up frequently during the night with difficulty returning to sleep, or waking up too early in the morning, or un-refreshing sleep.

**Insulin:** A natural hormone made by the pancreas that controls the level of sugar glucose in the blood. Insulin permits cells to use glucose for energy. Cells cannot utilize glucose without insulin.

**Insulin Resistance:** The diminished ability of cells to respond to the action of insulin in transporting glucose (sugar) from the bloodstream into muscle and other tissues. Insulin resistance typically develops with obesity and heralds the onset of Type 2 Diabetes. Insulin tries to access the muscle and the muscle accepts, but with insulin resistance, the muscle cannot acknowledge so the pancreas makes more insulin, which increases insulin levels in the blood. Eventually, the pancreas produces far more insulin than normal and the muscles continue to be resistant. Once the pancreas is no longer able to keep up, blood glucose starts to rise, initially after meals, eventually even in the fasting state. Type 2 Diabetes is now imminent.

**LAUP:** Laser assisted uvulopalatoplasty is surgery performed on the soft palate to reduce snoring (not recommended for sleep apnea).

**Mandible:** The bone of the lower jaw. The joint where the mandible meets the upper jaw at the temporal bone is called the temporomandibular joint.

**Maxilla:** The bone of the upper jaw.

**Metabolic:** Relating to metabolism, the whole range of biochemical processes that occur within us (or any living organism). Metabolism consists of anabolism (the buildup of substances) and catabolism (the breakdown of substances).

**Mixed Sleep Apnea:** A combination of obstructive (OSA) and central (CSA) sleep apnea.

**NREM:** Non Rapid Eye Movement sleep.

**Nasal passage:** A channel for airflow through the nose.

**Nasal Septum:** The divider between the left and right nose cavities made up of bone and cartilage and soft tissue (what you break when you have a broken nose).

**Obese:** What you are when your weight is in excess of 20% of your ideal body weight or Body Mass Index (BMI) in excess of 30.

**OSA:** Obstructive sleep apnea which is a breathing disorder characterized by brief interruptions of breathing during sleep. It owes its name to a Greek word, apnea, meaning "want of breath."

**Otolaryngologist:** An ear, nose and throat (ENT) specialist.

**Pharyngeal:** Having to do with the pharynx (throat).

**Pharynx:** The hollow tube that is about 5 inches long and starts behind the nose and ends at the top of the trachea (windpipe) and esophagus. The pharynx serves as an entry for the trachea and esophagus.

**PSG:** This is a polysomnograph or sleep test usually done in a sleep clinic.

**Polysomnography:** Continuous recording of specific physiologic variables during sleep, it typically records brain wave changes (electroencephalogram), eye movements (electrooculogram), muscle tone (electromyogram) respiration, electrocardiogram (EKG), and leg movements.

**Pulmonary:** Having to do with the lungs.

**Reflux:** The term used when liquid backs up into the esophagus from the stomach.

**REM Sleep**: This is the portion of sleep when there are rapid eye movements usually associated with dreams (REMs).

**Snoring:** A loud noise made on inspiration during sleep by vibration of the soft palate (the back of the roof of the mouth) and the uvula (the structure dangling down at the back of the mouth).

**Soft Palate:** The muscular part of the roof of the mouth. The soft palate is directly behind the hard palate, and it lacks bone.

**Stroke:** Sudden death of brain cells due to lack of oxygen, caused by blockage of blood flow or rupture of an artery to the brain. Sudden loss of speech, weakness, or paralysis of one side of the body can be symptoms. A suspected stroke can be confirmed by scanning the brain with special X-ray tests, such as CAT scans. The death rate and level of disability resulting from strokes can be dramatically reduced by immediate and appropriate medical care. Prevention involves minimizing risk such as controlling high blood pressure and diabetes.

**TMJ:** Temporomandibular joint (upper/lower jaw hook up here)

**Tonsillectomy:** The surgical removal of both tonsils.

**Tonsils:** Small masses of lymphoid tissue at the back and on both sides of the throat.

**Trachea:** A tube-like portion of the respiratory tract that connects the larynx with the bronchial parts of the lungs. Also known as windpipe.

**Upper Airway Resistance Syndrome (UARS):** A type of sleep-disordered breathing associated with arousals from sleep.

**Uvula:** The anatomic structure that dangles downward at the back of the mouth and is attached to the rear of the soft palate.

**UPPP:** This is an uvulopalatopharyngoplasty which is a type of operation designed to tighten up flabby tissues and enlarge the upper air passages. The operation involves reshaping the uvula, soft palate and throat.

# Chapter Three

## A History of the Study of Sleep Apnea

Although there are references to what appears to be sleep apnea in ancient East Indian and European mythologies, experts can probably agree that the Charles Dickens work called Pickwick Papers penned in 1827 may be the first time a clear description of this affliction was articulated. A website on Dickens (perryweb.com/dickens) describes it this way:

Obesity Hypoventilation Syndrome (OHS), a condition related to sleep apnea, was first called *"Pickwickian Syndrome."* It's named after the book because the novel features a character with all the classic symptoms as described like this:

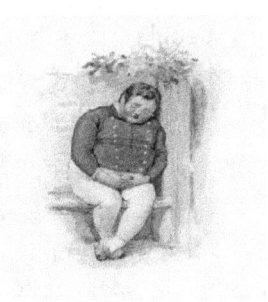

*The object that presented itself to the eyes of the astonished clerk, was a boy—a wonderfully fat boy-habited as a serving lad, standing upright on the mat, with his eyes closed as if in sleep. Joe is constantly hungry, very red in the face and is always falling asleep in the middle of tasks.*

*...on the box sat a fat and red-faced boy, in a state of somnolency...*

*..."damn that boy;" said the old gentleman, "he's gone to sleep again."*

*"Sleep!" said the old gentleman, 'he's always asleep. Goes on errands fast asleep, and snores as he waits at table." How very odd!" said Mr. Pickwick.*

*"Ah! Odd indeed," returned the old gentleman; "I'm proud of that boy-wouldn't part with him on any account-he's a natural curiosity!"*

OHS occurs when severely overweight people don't breathe rapidly enough or deeply enough. The lack of proper breathing leads to the oxygen levels in their blood being low and the carbon dioxide levels being too high. Some people with OHS also develop sleep apnea. People with sleep apnea stop breathing for short times while they're sleeping. This disruptive pattern can occur many times during a single night and can put a strain on the heart.

People with OHS and sleep apnea can be very drowsy during the day and fall asleep during inappropriate times. Sleep apnea makes people tired because of the lack of a good night's sleep. OHS causes sleepiness because of the high levels of carbon dioxide in the blood.

In 1956 a poker-playing businessman developed similar symptoms to the character *Joe* of *The Pickwick Papers*. People studying his condition named it "Pickwickian Syndrome" because in describing *Joe*, Dickens had perfectly described the main symptoms of the condition. Here's a quote from the original study:

*Finally an experience which indicated the severity of his disability led him to seek hospital care. The patient was accustomed to playing poker once a week and on this crucial occasion he was dealt a hand of three aces and two kings. According to Hoyle this hand is called a 'full house.'*

*Because he had dropped off to sleep he failed to take advantage of this opportunity. A few days later he entered hospital.*

Dickens would no doubt have appreciated the humor in the medical report. It's now more common to use the term OHS to refer to this condition. If you drive for a living and think you may have the symptoms described here, **get yourself tested!**

It wasn't until the mid 1950s that sleep apnea was even considered a medical condition when concerned scientists actually began observing people with unexplained medical issues while they were asleep. In the hundred or so years up to that point, they had always concluded that some virus or bacteria was the underlying cause of what ailed them. This was the beginning of sleep testing, later referred to as polysomnography.

They soon realized that sleep is not necessarily peaceful, and that led to the new science of sleep medicine. Patients began to get treated for the sleep disorder itself as opposed to treating the damage it caused, like heart disease and diabetes for example.

It is only since the late 1970s and early 1980s that it has been finally recognized for what it is, a serious medical health problem. Notwithstanding, the average non-medical person has no idea just how serious, nor does that person fathom how many other illnesses it is associated with. Sleep apnea is still not readily identified by family doctors as their mindset is still geared to treating the results of having sleep apnea, and not the sleep apnea itself.

# The Three Classifications of Sleep Disorders

This book is not about sleep disorders in general. However, you can explore them further by reading Sleep Disorders for Dummies, or here is a rundown on what the main ones are because treating them in the conventional manner can actually worsen a person with sleep apnea. The message is the same though, if you're on the road driving for a living then **get tested!**

The list of sleep disorders recognized by the medical community is now over 70. In America it is reported that about 40 million people suffer from a chronic sleep disorder, while around 20 million more suffer from occasional sleep difficulties. This list of sleep disorders is divided into three categories:

1) *Disturbed Sleep* (insomnia)
2) *Excessive Sleep* (hypersomnia)
3) *Lack of Sleep* (sleep deprivation)

Once a sleep disorder is diagnosed, there are treatment options. However, often people are unaware of their sleep disorder until a spouse or another person observes their sleep. Sleep disorders vary with causes, symptoms and frequency. Variances are in how long it takes to fall asleep, the quality of one's sleep, and how long one sleeps.

# A List of Other Sleep Disorders

**Insomnia:** *Difficulty falling asleep and staying asleep. It can be a temporary sleep condition or develop into a more chronic long term sleep disorder.*

**Hypersomnia:** *The opposite of insomnia. A person sleeps longer and for more hours than what is normal - during the night or the day. It is difficult for them to wake up. The need to take naps is compelling, but provides no relief.*

**Bedwetting:** *Another name is sleep enuresis which is bed-wetting while sleeping.*

**Bruxism:** *Clenching and grinding the teeth while sleeping. This condition is common in children but also occurs in adults.*

**Cataplexy**: *Abrupt weakness with one's motor muscles.*

**Delayed Sleep Phase Syndrome (DSPS):** *Fall asleep and waken at unusual times, but able to maintain sleep (circadian rhythms disorder)*

**Advanced Sleep Phase Syndrome (ASPS):** *Another circadian rhythms disorder where a person goes to sleep early and rises early*

**Non-24-Hour Sleep-Wake Syndrome**: *Circadian rhythm disorder where the body does not function with the 24 hour biological clock.*

**Hypopnea Syndrome**: *A slow respiratory rate or shallow breathing while sleeping.*

**Narcolepsy**: *Unwilling and spontaneous falling asleep with excessive daytime sleepiness*

**Night Terror**: *Not nightmares but rather a sudden awakening with gasping, moaning, or crying out. There is no recall of the episode in the morning. It is not uncommon in young children, but adults can experience it as well.*

**Nocturia**: *A recurring need to go to the bathroom and urinate at night.*

**Parasomnia**: *Arousal disorder with abnormal behaviors and thoughts such as sleep walking.*

**Restless Leg Syndrome (RLS)**: *Associated  Periodic Limb Movement with an irresistible need to move the leg.*

**Periodic Limb Movement Disorder (PLMD) / Nocturnal Mycolonus**: *The involuntary movement of legs and/or arms while sleeping.*

**Rapid Eye Movement Behavior Disorder (RBD)**: *Movements in REM sleep from twitches to acting out dreams.*

**Situational Circadian Rhythm Sleep Disorders**: *Jet lag and shift work sleep disorders (SWSD).*

**Sleep Paralysis**: *A temporal paralysis of the body right before or after sleep. Often associated with auditory, visual, or tactile hallucinations. Sometimes classified as a part of narcolepsy.*

**Sleep Walking / Somnambulism**: *Doing actions typical with being awake such as walking around, eating or dressing, without conscious knowledge or awareness.*

**Snoring**: *It is a symptom of a problem and not an actual disorder*

**Sleeping Sickness:** *Parasite disease transmitted by the Tsetse fly*

**Sleep Talking / Somniloquy:** *Talking while sleeping*

**Sudden Infant Death Syndrome (SIDS):** *The sudden death of an infant under the age of one. It usually occurs in the crib while the baby is sleeping.*

## A Personal Story of Sleep Apnea and Narcolepsy (and Being Reported to the Authorities)

There are one or two sleep disorders that capture the attention of transportation authorities, maybe even more so than sleep apnea.

*Clearly, narcolepsy and cataplexy are terms you do not want to be associated with if you drive for a living.* Just review the definitions above and it will become clear as to why.

I'm a little ahead of the section that discusses treatment options, but while on the subject of sleep disorders this seemed like the right time to discuss this. As professional drivers, I know that loss of license is the issue that is front and centre. Aside from the personal cost of treatment options, it is the number one reason that there are literally thousands of you on the road with undiagnosed sleep apnea.

I have been successfully treated for my sleep apnea for about 16 years now with the use of an oral appliance fitted by a dentist trained in Sleep Therapy. In 2010, I went for another sleep test at a sleep clinic for two reasons. Firstly, I weighed about 30 lbs more than my previous sleep test in 1995 and wanted to see what the severity of my sleep apnea was all these years later. Secondly, I had never tried or even considered a CPAP device and wanted to try it out for myself before I could write about it credibly. Why not? The $2500 cost of the best unit with all the bells and whistles was covered by my health plan to the tune of about $1800 leaving only about $700 coming from my pocket.

The results of the sleep test were horrific while sleeping without my oral device. My readings were in the 'severe apnea' category, which was somewhat predictable with the weight I was carrying and a neck size of over 17 inches. The sleep doctor provided me with a CPAP machine for one month to try out before adopting it as my own. During that time, I found that I could fall asleep with it on if I was good and tired, but if I woke up for any reason it was impossible to get back to sleep. So I would discard it and insert my oral appliance for the rest of the night.

Later, I went for another follow-up sleep test at the same lab, only this time I went to sleep with the CPAP and no oral appliance. I was wired up and in bed by 11 PM with a plan for the lab staff to wake me about 5 AM to send me home.

Between 11 PM and 1 AM the technician repeatedly came into my room because they could tell I was unable to sleep (they would know since I was being electronically monitored). It was pointless, so I got up in bed, shut down the CPAP (knowing they would be rebounding into the room any second) and when they got there I announced that I was going home to sleep and asked if they would kindly remove the probes stuck all over my body.

I can tell you this was not looked upon kindly. I am not sure how often this happened to them, but I was done. Of course, this would be reported to the sleep doctor the next day who interpreted my behavior as flat out rejecting treatment for a severe sleep apnea.

In his mind, the sleep doctor was obliged to report me to the Department of Transport, which he did. You should be aware at this point that every state, province, jurisdiction, etc., has this rule. It not only applies to commercial drivers, but to anyone who holds a valid driver's license. Understandably, they don't want us out there killing innocent people as well as ourselves while making a mess all over their roadways, which they have to clean up at their expense.

I have a commercial driver's license even though I was not using it at the time to earn a living. Nevertheless, I am not into taking public transit or taxis, so I needed my license to get around just as much as any commercial driver needs it to earn a living.

Not to digress, but I was not even thinking he would report me because he knew that I had been using an oral device for years to mitigate my sleep apnea, which brings me to the next point about reporting.

Most doctors in most jurisdictions will report you to reduce their own legal and medical exposure. The rules tend to be somewhat vague from place to place in terms of what is required of them, so you can probably count on being reported. The good news is, the transport people will write you and give you time to be treated. The sleep doctor who reports you will immediately confirm on your behalf that you are under treatment (sort of). In fact, my sleep doctor would not have reported me at all had I not left the sleep lab. Had I completed the test proving that the CPAP successfully treated my sleep apnea, it would not have been an issue at all.

But there is much more to the story. The sleep doctor met with me and accepted my plea that I never should have been reported once I again made it clear that all I was doing was trying out a CPAP unit. He then sent another *form letter* to the transport people in an attempt to reverse the error, but the letter included the pre-printed words "Sleep Apnea/Narcolepsy" that implied that I had one or the other (he simply circled 'sleep apnea') as his way of telling them all is right with my personal situation. The government people however, wanted to know all the details about my "Narcolepsy"" which I did NOT have!

To unravel that crisis, I had to go to both my personal doctor and my dentist to get written proof that I was diagnosed in the mid-

90s as having a moderate to severe sleep apnea that has been successfully treated with an oral device. To further prove my innocence, my dentist provided me with his *Embletta X100* portable sleep test machine to sleep with my oral device inserted. This unit does everything that can be achieved in the sleep clinic except measure the various sleep levels (not critical in determining whether you have sleep apnea or not). The results then have to be downloaded and sent to a qualified sleep specialist to be read and interpreted. A dentist can treat you, but only after a diagnosis by a qualified sleep specialist. A dentist cannot diagnose.

I did that in addition to having my personal doctor write to the government. Meanwhile, I had the original sleep specialist (the doctor who caused the problem in the first place) send another letter, which his administrative assistant allowed me to edit (remove any reference to narcolepsy) before submitting. I think she helped me out in that regard because she recognized the unfairness of the situation. I recommended to her that in future to stop using form letters or this will keep on happening.

I fully understand the trepidation professional drivers have when it comes to hiding a sleep disorder, but you will read later on that there is much more to the issue. You may eventually kill yourself by not seeking help, and it may not be on the road. There are myriad health issues associated with sleep apnea. Aside from that, there is a moral issue whereby you will hurt others in the process of ignoring your own health. In all likelihood you will affect your own family and friends in addition to the strangers you inadvertently involve in a highway accident. Keep reading and plan on getting yourself evaluated.

## Every Living Animal Needs to Sleep

American Journalist David Randall wrote a book called *Dreamland: Adventures in the Strange Science of Sleep,* which was released in August 2012. He was motivated by his penchant for sleepwalking that started about three years earlier. That month he did an interview with Brian Bethune for Maclean's magazine and the highlights of that interview follow.

His doctor offered up some sleeping pills. Randall figured there is not much anybody *really* knows about sleep, but that he could do better than that. For something that the population spends approximately one-third of their lives doing and has since the beginning of time, why do we know so little about it? Worse, why is it that the sleep medication market size is over $30 Billion? It is what it is because it's a function of treating the results of sleep issues versus focusing on getting to the cause by way of a polysomnogram (or PSG).

We don't even know why we and every other animal sleeps in the first place given the fact that we are effectively shut down while there are predators all around us. Most hoofed animals sleep about an hour and a half or less per day – probably for that reason. Yet the impact of sleep is profound since studies show that sleep is more important than what you eat, or even your income. It cannot be argued, with everything you do during the day you can show the impact sleep has on it. Sleep is now thought of as one of the absolute best forms of preventative medicine. Did you know that sleep is one of the biggest parts of training an Olympic athlete?

You are driving a truck or a bus, not exactly a 9 to 5 job. It is virtually equal to working rotating shifts. A recent study found a 74 percent spike in breast cancer rates among nurses working the night shift. They rotate days to afternoons to overnights and back, and their bodies never get into a rhythm so they are negatively impacted on a cellular level. They do not get enough melatonin from natural daylight that is essential to the healing process, and they do this for 25 to 35 years? The experts postulate that these rotating shifts are the worst form of sleep hygiene, and that consistency in sleep is probably much more important than the hours slept.

Another study of medical interns who often work stretches of 30 hours, show them as functioning well at their jobs, but not so well outside of them. You can be sleep deprived and adjust to it because you are able to adequately anticipate what is required of you as you carry out your work. But then they leave work and have horrible accident rates. It can be argued that your driving job does not equate to the action going on at the typical emergency ward at a hospital. Let's face it, most of the time you're on cruise control.

Fatigue management is becoming big business now. Companies are realizing it's a global marketplace so the potential to do business these days is literally around the clock. The smarter companies are implementing fatigue control policies where they enforce mandatory break times, and those companies who do random testing of employees to really ensure employees are awake are the companies whose accident costs are plummeting. Companies like Google and Nike have nap strategies because they do not want to lose staff to Apple or Yahoo, so they allow their employees to sleep more and take naps on the job. Do you expect that to happen with professional drivers and the transportation companies they work for? Not quite the same way, so you have to take matters into your own hands and deal with your own potential sleep apnea. You already know if you're a candidate.

Dawn, daylight, dusk and dark are what influence your circadian rhythms. Once you've established them, that is what makes you go to sleep naturally and wake up without an alarm clock.

Did you know that in the history of Monday Night Football, when all other variables are accounted for like injuries and weather, West Coast teams playing East Coast teams have won 70 percent of the games? They feel like they are playing after a typical day shift job when they get that bolt of energy around dinner time. Meanwhile, the East Coast team is tired out by 10 PM.

Maybe you can see now why Olympic level athletes incorporate sleep hygiene as an equal part of their overall training. A long haul trucker and/or OTR bus driver will seldom enjoy a healthy routine when it comes to sleep; so all the more reason to carry on reading, absorb the material then get yourself tested.

# Chapter Four

## What is Sleep Apnea Exactly?

*Sleep Apnea* is a condition whereby you cease to breathe during sleep. When you stop breathing, that is the actual apnea occurring. The word is Greek and literally means "the cessation of breath." When you fail to totally stop breathing, or when the cessation is incomplete or is shallow breathing (meaning there is a substantial reduction in the intake of air), that is called *Hypopnea.* For it to be determined that you have sleep apnea or hypopnea, the complete or partial cessation of breathing must be at least 10 seconds in length. The actual term 'sleep apnea' encompasses both apneas and hypopneas.

## Normal Sleep versus Sleep Apnea Breathing

Normal sleep breathing for an adult is rhythmic and consists of about 12 breaths per minute. Each breath is about the same inhalation depth with a slight pause between inhaling and exhaling. This pattern lasts quite awhile before the sleeper takes a deeper breath and repositions himself in bed.

Sleep apnea breathing on the other hand is labored and much faster when it is actually happening. The depth of each breath is often inconsistent with the one before. Also, usually included in the pattern are incidents of no breathing at all. During this time there is almost always shifting of position, head movement, and moaning or other sounds. The depth of a breath generally becomes more shallow just before it ceases altogether momentarily. Some have no pre-gasp breath but instead go directly from no breathing to a sudden large gasp, which frequently awakens them completely. The apnea often gets worse later in the night during the time when REM level sleep generally occurs. This is the time during your sleep when you recharge yourself, but instead you tend to awaken un-rested and most frequently with your blood pressure elevated.

## What Are the Types of Sleep Apnea?

There are two main types plus a hybrid of both to make a total of three. About 90% of those diagnosed with sleep apnea will have what is known as *Obstructive Sleep Apnea* (OSA) which is characterized by an ongoing physical obstruction of the upper airway. The other main type is called *Central Sleep Apnea* (CSA) which makes up the other 10% of those diagnosed. It is neurological in nature and is literally a failure of the brain to tell you to breathe. The third type is called 'Mixed Sleep Apnea' and is a combination of CSA and OSA, usually beginning as CSA then becoming OSA. There are other sub-types like *Upper Airway Resistance Syndrome* (UARS) and *Obesity Hypoventilation Syndrome* (OHS) as described earlier as the character 'Joe' in Dickens' work The Pickwick Papers.

## How Does OHS Differ from OSA?

OHS is considered an extreme version of OSA although it is a little more detailed than that. OHS diagnosed patients are always obese while OSA patients are as a rule, but not necessarily so. OSA patients generally do not retain carbon dioxide during the day while OHS patients do. OSA *may* lead to hypertension where it does not already exist, while OHS almost always will.

# How Common is OSA?

Go back to Chapter 2 and read the definition again for AHI. It is at least as common as diabetes and asthma. As the prevalence of obesity skyrockets in western society with both our aging population and with the younger generation stuck in front of television, video games and the Internet, there is no ceiling to where this epidemic is going. Sitting at the wheel of a truck or bus for 10 or so hours a day is just as bad. If you have an AHI higher than five as do about 25% of adult males and about 10% of adult women, then you may be on your way.

# How is Snoring Related?

Snoring is one of the main clinical differences between OSA and CSA. Part and parcel of snoring are witnessed apneas (ask the person you sleep with), choking and gasping for air, repeatedly waking up (arousals), excessive daytime sleepiness, apparent sleep but never really rested, overall physically fatigued all the time, headaches when you awaken, apparent mood disorders, and finally impotence (who knew that?).

Snoring is essentially 'noisy breathing' during sleep, and is the sound caused due to the vibration of the soft tissue at the back of your throat and/or air turbulently passing through the nose. Snoring does not automatically mean you have sleep apnea, however virtually all those with diagnosed sleep apnea do snore. If you snore but do not have diagnosed sleep apnea yet, this is known as primary snoring. Snoring should be regarded as a 'red flag' for sleep apnea, especially if you snore loud enough to rearrange the bedroom furniture and keep others from sleeping. If you have daytime sleepiness and blood pressure averaging over 140/90, you are on your way and you should be tested.

To be clear, snoring is not an illness in and of itself. On some levels it is simply a social inconvenience, but it is a medical symptom for sure. It could simply be a result of the common cold or a variety of allergies, but it does interfere with normal breathing. Really healthy people tend to breathe through their nose on the basis that they have sufficient space in their throat to allow air to flow. As we age we not only get fat on the outside, but also on the inside as things evolve. If you've ever breathed into a paper or plastic bag, you can clearly see it collapse as you watch the resulting vacuum effect. Your throat is also collapsible, and although it doesn't totally cave in it gets pretty violent in there as you try to breathe.

## When Does Snoring Become Abnormal?

When snoring lasts longer than about 10 seconds or so, the oxygen in your red blood cells begins to decrease. This is called hypopnea and is easily diagnosed by a pulse oximeter during a polysomnogram (PSG or Sleep Test). Your oxygen level should always be 90 percent at a minimum. When it drops below that, it is called oxygen desaturization because you have had either a hypopneic or apneic event. When you add the number of both of these events together over a one hour period, this establishes the index by which you are assessed. A severe sleep apnea occurs beginning at 30 RDI (respiratory disturbance index) or 30 AHI (these terms are becoming somewhat interchangeable). All those who snore do not necessarily have OSA, but they may have OSH or UARS (Upper Airway Resistance Syndrome).

# What Are Some of the Causes?

You can be genetically predisposed, but if you are you are more likely to find that out during your earlier growth years. For the average person, especially those who work a relatively sedentary job like driving for a living, and who live a rather sedentary lifestyle overall, obesity is a key indicator and age 40 seems to be the age where it will become an undeniable issue. Just think about the typical 'truck stop diet' too, and just how many professional drivers still tend to smoke cigarettes.

In terms of measuring obesity, the *Body Mass Index* (BMI) tends to be referred to most often although there are better ways to categorize obesity. For example, a BMI greater than 25 indicates a person is fat and a BMI greater than 30 suggests they are obese. Some say if your weight exceeds 20% of your charted ideal weight you are obese. Have you ever seen one of those insurance charts for males and/or females that say a certain height should equal a certain weight? Arguably they are idiotic and fail to take the three body types (esomorph, endomorph, ectomorph) into consideration. I think a fairer measurement is a waist size over 40 inches for men, and over 34 inches for women combined with a neck size over 17 inches for men and 16 inches for women. Take the obesity factor and add one or more of these considerations:

1) Are you an aging male or a pre/post menopausal woman?
2) Are you a smoker?
3) Do you have a craniofacial deformity?
4) Do you have enlarged adenoids and tonsils?
5) Do you have a deviated septum?
6) Do you have chronic nasal congestion?
7) Are you a user of alcohol and sedatives?
8) Do you have an endocrine disorder?
9) And finally, what is your family history?

Make no mistake, if you want to begin to deal with your snoring and sleep disorder issue (diagnosed or undiagnosed), lose fat. The number one source of all that ails us in 2013 is obesity. Almost everything else that is wrong with us starts right there. Obstructive sleep apnea is no different.

# Chapter Five

## Just How Serious is Untreated Sleep Apnea?

In the case of a professional truck or bus driver, the most obvious risk is of a traffic accident potentially severely injuring or killing yourself, other innocent drivers, and both yours and their passengers. You are at least fifteen times higher risk of accident both on the road and elsewhere in the workplace. That should be incentive enough to get checked out, but it gets worse. *Here is a list of medical conditions associated with sleep apnea:*

- *Heart Disease (risk is x 20)*
- *Irregular Heartbeat (arrhythmia)*
- *Stroke (risk is x3)*
- *Coronary Artery Disease*
- *Cerebrovascular Disease*
- *Congestive Heart Failure*
- *Hypertension*
- *Diabetes Mellitus*
- *Excessive Sleepiness*
- *Obesity (uncontrolled weight gain)*
- *Bi-polarism*
- *Acid Reflux (GERD)*
- *Depression*
- *Severe Headaches*
- *Cancer*
- *Impotence (ED)*
- *Irritability*
- *Memory Loss*

No doubt you've heard of *Sudden Infant Death Syndrome* (SIDS), or more commonly referred to as Crib Death in babies usually less than a year old. Sleep apnea is almost always suspected as the real cause.

You often hear of people simply dying in their sleep from 'natural causes.' Sleep apnea is also frequently suspected when this occurs.

Sleep apnea and sleep disorders in general can dramatically weaken your immune system. It has been proven in laboratory animals that tumors can grow two to three times faster with severe sleep dysfunctions present. It also impairs production of melatonin which is a hormone and potent anti-oxidant that usually retains cancer fighting properties.

Sleep apnea can cause a pre-diabetic state that makes you feel hungry even after a meal, and that initiates uncontrollable weight gain. It also contributes to stomach ulcers, constipation, memory loss, problem solving abilities and mood disorders like depression.

If you manage to escape all that, did you know that seniors with sleep apnea appear to have more than twice the odds of developing dementia years later? So do those who develop disruptions of their circadian rhythm (typically shift workers and those with work schedules like professional drivers).

The bottom line is, you'll probably just die at an age much earlier than had to be. All this because you either failed to recognize that you were afflicted, or you did know you were a likely candidate for diagnosed sleep apnea, but did nothing about it.

Sleep apnea is highly treatable and the best results will occur before you cause any further residual damage. Get yourself tested!

## Co-Morbidity and Co-existing Disease Factors

Working backwards, people who have been diagnosed with certain medical conditions are often *later* found to have sleep apnea. To the same extent, those already diagnosed with sleep apnea are likely to develop certain future medical complications. Look at these rates of co-morbidity and decide if you are a candidate to make yourself even sicker:

- Hypertension       40 – 50%

- Coronary heart disease       34%

- Congestive heart failure       34%

- Diabetes       65%

- Erectile dysfunction       50%

- Renal disease       50%

- Fibromyalgia       80%

- Nocturnal strokes       84%

There is also a high correlation between patients who have Gastroesophageal Reflux (GERD)) and OSA. As far as diabetes is concerned, excessive apneic events affect the production of insulin which encourages the onset of Type 2 Diabetes. These events also affect the permeability of the lining of your arteries by increasing the buildup of plaque and the chance of cardiovascular complications such as a heart attack. The weakening of the walls of your arteries then increases the susceptibility of rupturing of these vessels, and that is how you end up experiencing a stroke.

If you are a male, this affliction will capture your attention for sure. ***There is a direct correlation between OSA and erectile*** *dysfunction (ED)*. Scientists suspect this may have to do with sex hormones like testosterone which rise with sleep and fall when there is a lack of it. Therefore, intermittent waking and chronic sleep deprivation drives down these hormones usually causing sexual dysfunction.

In a recent study published in The Journal of Sexual Medicine, scientists compared 80 women with obstructive sleep apnea between the ages of 28 and 64 with 240 women without the condition. They found that the apnea patients had significantly higher rates of sexual dysfunction. In a study in 2009, researchers looked for signs of sexual problems in 401 men who showed up at a clinic for suspected sleep apnea. Of those who received an OSA diagnosis, about 70 percent also had erectile dysfunction compared with 34 percent in those without sleep apnea. On the bright side treatment can make a difference, but the bottom line is that sleep apnea still can raise the risk of sexual dysfunction.

Another study suggests *sleep apnea is associated with mental decline and dementia*. Published in The Journal of the American Medical Association, they studied 298 physically and mentally healthy women who completed a battery of tests of mental acuity as they spent a night attached to devices to measure breathing and wake-sleep patterns. Of the 298 women, 105 met the criteria for sleep-disordered breathing, with an average of 15 or more episodes of interrupted breathing per hour during the night (only mild OSA).

Five years later, 45 percent of the women with sleep-disordered breathing had developed mild cognitive impairment or dementia compared with 31 percent of those who slept normally. After controlling for age, race, body mass index, education level, smoking status, the presence of diabetes, hypertension, the use of antidepressants and other medicines, the women with sleep-disordered breathing at the start of the study were 85 percent more likely to have mild cognitive impairment or dementia after five years than those whose night time breathing was normal.

*Sleep itself plays a role in the long-term memory* too as scientists suspect that frequent interruptions of sleep and less sleep overall might cause the effect of losing it. They found that the number of sleep disruptions and the total duration of sleep had no association with mental impairment, rather it was the hypoxia or reduced oxygen to the brain caused by the breathing disruptions that was consistently associated with mental impairment. Studies suggest that if you treat sleep apnea you actually may improve cognitive ability. There is much wrong with ignoring the signs.

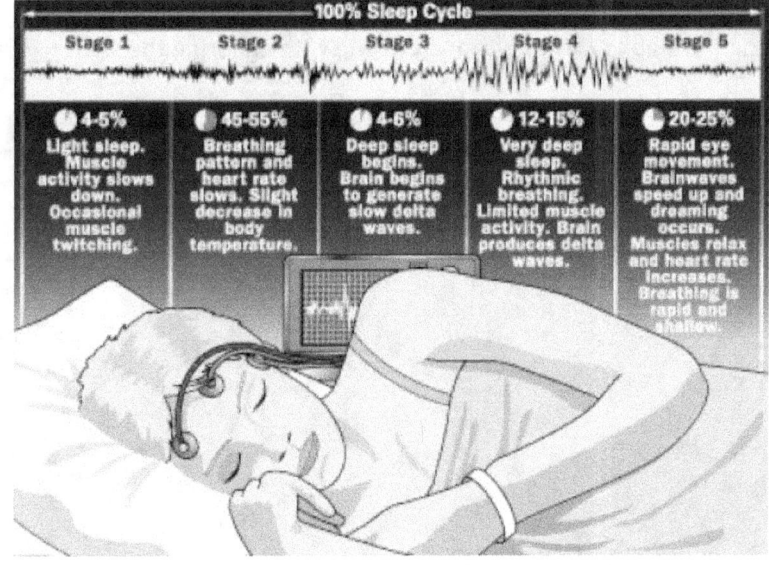

# Chapter Six

## Self-Diagnosis versus Proper Medical Diagnosis

I would only advocate starting with a self-diagnosis exercise because generally you know when something is amiss when it comes to your own health. You may not know exactly what is wrong, but you certainly know intuitively that for the multitude of reasons already identified, as a professional driver you are personally and morally required to get properly tested. However, you can start with a self-administered exercise called the Epworth Sleepiness Scale.

This test was created in 1991 by a doctor at Epworth Hospital in Melbourne Australia and it is simply in the format of a questionnaire. All it does is ask you to rate your probability of falling asleep on a scale of 0 to 3 for eight different situations that you encounter most days. You then add the scores for the eight questions together to obtain a single result. A result from 0 to 9 is considered to be normal, but a result in the 10–24 range indicates that expert medical advice should be sought. For instance, scores of 11-15 are shown to indicate the possibility of mild to moderate sleep apnea, where a score of 16 and above indicates the possibility of severe sleep apnea (or even narcolepsy).

Since you are self-administering the test, refrain from totaling your result after each question until you're done. Otherwise, you might sub-consciously affect your next answer. Don't cheat yourself - for now no one will see the outcome but you. However, once you seek a formal diagnosis this same test will very likely again be the very first step in the process. You will already know the outcome provided you are honest with yourself.

While you're doing that, give this test to someone who regularly observes you sleeping. The following questions relate to the behavior they observe. Choose the most appropriate number for each situation.

**0** = *Never*                     **1** = *Infrequently (once per week)*
**2** = *Frequently (2-3 nights)*   **3** = *Most of the time*

- Loud, irritating snoring _____

- Choking or gasping for air _____

- Pauses in breathing _____

- Twitching / kicking of arms or legs _____

- Snoring requiring separate bedrooms _____

- Falling asleep inappropriately_____

Add them up. A score of 5 or greater indicates symptoms which are affecting your health, safety, or quality of life. Give this result and your Epworth result to your doctor or dentist and get properly diagnosed and treated.

Finally, prioritize this list *from your personal perspective* (rank in order of what bothers you the most) to go with the above test and the one that follows. Give all three to your doctor.

| | | | |
|---|---|---|---|
| Frequent heavy snoring | ( ) | Affecting others sleep | ( ) |
| Daytime drowsiness | ( ) | Stop breathing when asleep | ( ) |
| Can't fall asleep | ( ) | Gasp for air when waking | ( ) |
| Choking at night | ( ) | Un-refreshed in the morning | ( ) |
| Wake up with headaches | ( ) | Wake up with hoarseness | ( ) |
| Grinding teeth at night | ( ) | Swelling in ankles or feet | ( ) |
| Jaw or facial pain | ( ) | Jaw clicking | ( ) |

Other concern:_____

# Epworth Sleepiness Scale

Name: _____     Today's Date: _____

Your Age (Years): _____     Your Sex (M/F): _____

How likely are you to *doze off* or *fall asleep* in the following situations in contrast to simply feeling tired? This refers to your usual way of life in recent times. Even if you haven't done some of these things recently, try to work out how they would have affected you. Use the following scale to choose the **most appropriate number** for each situation:

0 = would **never** doze          1 = **slight chance** of dozing
2 = **moderate chance** of dozing    3 = **high chance** of dozing

*It is important that you answer each question as best you can.*

### Situational Chance of Dozing (0-3)

1. Sitting and reading                                    (   )
2. Watching TV                                           (   )
3. Sitting, inactive in a public place or meeting        (   )
4. As a passenger in a car for an hour without a break   (   )
5. Lying down to rest in the afternoon                   (   )
6. Sitting and talking to someone                        (   )
7. Sitting quietly after a lunch without alcohol         (   )
8. In a car, while stopped for a few minutes in the traffic  (   )

*Total*          ____

*Developed by Dr. M.W. Johns 1990-97*

There is similar test called the Berlin Sleep Questionnaire if you really need further self-proof before seeing a doctor. If you are reading the eBook click Berlin Sleep Questionnaire, otherwise just open your browser and type in the address http://apnea-snoring.com/berlin_sleep_questions.html to see the test and to also find yourself a BMI Calculator.

If you go to the Apple App Store there are all sorts of different sleep test apps and BMI calculators there for free. In fact, there is a Sleep Medicine Test for physicians there for $150. This is serious business now!

## Pros and Cons of Self-Diagnosis

Based on the evidence, it's probably not hard to conclude that you have some sort of a sleep disorder, but is it a result of something else, or is it actually the catalyst for everything that ails you? Sleep apnea is seemingly omnipresent, but you might have something else wrong altogether (see the previous section on Sleep Disorders).

You could have a heart condition, a neurological disorder, or a breathing problem that is confused with sleep apnea. Just as easily, you could miss the fact that you have sleep apnea at all because of other medications you might be taking, including sedatives and alcohol. Or it could be related to depression and who knows what else?

The point is, it would *not* be hard to misdiagnose and self-prescribe the wrong treatment. Or worse, not be diagnosed at all. The Epworth exercise you just did is a good start, but it is not accurate enough to distinguish one sleep disorder from another. It is also very subjective, so relying on the results of it alone could easily cause you to under-estimate (or even over-estimate) severity. The only reason I mention it at all is to simply get you off your behind to start dealing with your personal situation before you really hurt yourself.

Even detailed testing (PSG) done in a hospital or sleep lab can result in a misdiagnosis for lots of reasons. For instance, some people cannot relax enough on the first try to duplicate the sleep conditions you usually experience, therefore the results may not be reflective of your reality.

Secondly, there are differences between daytime and night time sleep characteristics, not to mention the differences between sleep quality in the first half of the night versus the second half of the night. Remember too, this is a relatively new medical specialty (art) and most regular doctors don't have a clue when it comes to these diagnoses. A diagnosis must be done by a doctor where sleep medicine or sleep therapy is their specialty.

Not to discount your own family doctor, but don't assume he knows what he doesn't know about this subject. If you think you have an issue, by all means start there, but ask him to refer you to a specialist. Better yet, get him to arrange an appointment for you at an accredited sleep test center for a polysomnogram, the results of which are always given to a specialist to interpret.

## A Self-Diagnosis Option

If you are alone and no one has told you how bad your sleep characteristics are, try this in addition to the Epworth test. You can download an application (App) from ITunes or buy or borrow a Digital Voice Recorder. Most have enough memory for 20 hours or more, and you won't need that much. The idea is to record yourself snoring and holding your breath (apnea). Suspend the recorder near your head somehow, then go to sleep as usual after turning it on and ensuring the meter is registering the sound of your voice recording plus the date and time.

Most DVRs have a USB connector to plug into your computer, so downloading a file or two is easy. Later you can listen to yourself on your computer's sound system at high volume if you really want a wake-up call (pardon the analogy). Listening to the results can be a revelation and I can assure you that there is a high probability that you will become highly motivated to take the next step towards getting a sleep study done. Let your family doctor hear it for himself which will expedite a referral.

## A Primer on the Stages of Sleep

I alluded earlier to the *quantity* of sleep in terms of hours, but that has little to do with the *quality* of sleep required to reset yourself. Having a sleep disorder, perceived or otherwise, interferes with the reset process. Everybody is a little different in terms of their personal requirements, but there is no mistaking the difference between being 'un-rested' and unable to make it through the normal awake period, and waking up in an optimal frame of mind because you just had a great session of deep sleep. It truly is all in your head....or brain to be more accurate.

There are only <u>two kinds of sleep</u>: *Rapid Eye Movement (REM)* and *Non-Rapid Eye Movement (NREM).* There are <u>four stages</u> of *NREM plus REM* (the fifth stage).

Passing through all these stages takes about 90-110 minutes and marks one full sleep cycle. If you sleep soundly for eight hours per night, you're getting five full sleep cycles. Here is how it all happens:

**Stage 1:** *Light sleep, easily woken, begin to lose muscle tone, twitches and suddenly awake from dozing, loss of self awareness and most senses, brainwave frequencies descend from **ALPHA** through **THETA** state (4-7 Hz).*

**Stage 2:** *Loss of nearly all muscle tone so you can't act out dreams when they happen; brainwaves slowed further with bursts of higher brainwave activity (spindles) in the lower **BETA** range at 12-16 Hz (about half of all your sleep is Stage 2).*

**Stage 3:** *Begin deep sleep; hard to rouse, but if you do you will feel dopey/confused for a minute; brainwaves descended to **DELTA** range of 0.5-4 Hz (slowest frequency); dreamless but where sleepwalking occurs.*

**Stage 4:** *Is the Deepest Slow Wave Sleep; replenishes both physical/mental energy and without it you won't feel refreshed; brainwaves exclusively **DELTA**.*

**REM:** *Onset of dreams; after deep stages brainwaves return to the **THETA** through **BETA** range; if woken you return here when you next sleep; creation of long-term memories occur here; lucid dreaming; brainwaves sometimes **GAMMA** range of 38-90 Hz; highly active brain state.*

So, can you see the problem when your sleep pattern prevents you from getting enough deep stage sleep? When you have a successful sleep test (PSG) in a sleep lab, it will measure your sleep in this level of detail. If you have a home sleep test (like with the *Embletta X100*), it provides enough information for a qualified sleep specialist to diagnose a sleep disorder such as sleep apnea, but it does not provide the detail on your personal stages of sleep.

# Testing for Sleep Apnea

## The Polysomnogram (PSG) Experience

Whether you are referred to a hospital sleep clinic or a privately operated sleep lab, this is the highest standard testing for sleep apnea. Generally speaking, they tend to try to duplicate your usual sleeping environment at home by having you sleep in what appears to be a normal bedroom. Most labs consist of five to seven bedrooms but could be bigger or smaller. Regardless, the technicians must prepare an equal number of test subjects before sending you off to sleep for the night. In order to accomplish that, typically they will ask you to report at a specific time starting at around 9:00 PM until about 10:30 PM, at which point they will wire you with a multitude of sensors that are attached directly to your skin.

This process is not unlike having an routine ECG during your annual physical exam, nor is it really any different than being wired up for a lie detector test. They ask you to bring with you whatever attire you usually sleep in and you can even bring your own pillow (or teddy bear) if you like. You can probably have your iPod or a book to read if that makes you fall asleep easier, but check with the lab first. Washrooms are nearby for use in advance of the sleep test, or during the night if necessary, and for getting ready to leave in the morning. As a rule, they tend to wake you up around 5AM to 'unplug' you and send you on your way home.

Usually, they will have already scheduled you for a follow-up appointment with the sleep doctor to review the results and begin a course of treatment if required. It's a good idea to arrive for your sleep test good and tired since trying to sleep in unfamiliar surroundings sometimes keeps you alert for a period of time in excess of your normal routine at home. Sometimes this may skew the results. If you happen to be a nighthawk like me, I could probably lie there all night wide awake except I noticed they keep the room on the warm side to make sure you get drowsy more quickly.

There are as many as 16 sensors attached to your body in preparation for monitoring your sleep, but here are the main ones and their function:

1. *EEG (electroencephalogram) for brainwaves*

2. *ECG (electrocardiogram) for heart*

3. *Respiratory effort (nasal-oral air flow)*

4. *Arterial oxygen saturation (oximetry)*

5. *Tibial EMG leg movement sensor*

6. *Thoracic effort (motion) chest band sensor*

7. *Abdominal effort (motion) stomach band sensor*

8. *Body position (Left, Right and Supine)*

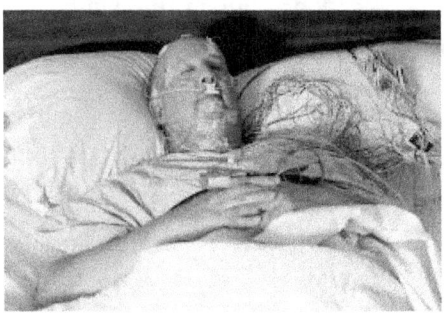 The collection of wires all go into a small computer-like casing or junction box that stays with you, but are tied off to keep everything out of the way. The data is automatically transferred to the main monitoring room where they keep an eye on you all night long and can make adjustments should any of the probes be faulty or otherwise fail to collect the necessary information. It's a little inconvenient but the process is totally painless.

The highest credential for a sleep lab technician is Registered Polysomnographic Technologist (RPST) and this person is responsible for attaining accurate results. A poorly conducted sleep test can result in a misdiagnosis and the wrong treatment, so don't be afraid to make sure the technician can demonstrate this. They do this every night and may be complacent about explaining what is going on, so feel free to make them work and get your money's worth by playing '20 Questions' if you feel so inclined.

Do your part of the preparation by avoiding caffeine, alcohol and taking cat-naps the day of your test (for obvious reasons). There will likely be an infrared camera recording you visually, a two-way speaker if you need to get up during the night so you can alert the technician, and there may be a separate microphone for purposes of recording your snoring which helps give perspective to the data collected. Just prior to going to sleep, the technician will test the equipment, so you will be asked to open and close your eyes, move them around, snore, take breaths in and out, and even move your arms and legs around. If something goes wrong with a wire, or if one comes loose during the night, your technician will come in to fix it.

If you get diagnosed with sleep apnea and are prescribed treatment, you can expect to be back in the lab at some future point to be tested again to measure the results, so get comfortable with the process.

## The Home Sleep Test Experience

Today with technological advancements, a PSG can be performed at home with fairly sophisticated but very portable equipment. After a briefing and instruction, the patient self-administers the home sleep test and is able to spend the night in their own bed in familiar surroundings. This is particularly advantageous to those whom are homebound, elderly, are experiencing chronic illness, or who require specialized care such as a nurse or family member spending the night. In some cases, it saves transportation costs.

The typical cost of a home sleep test is minute compared to the cost of an in-lab sleep test, and typically yields similar results in the diagnosis of Obstructive Sleep Apnea. Most times when a home sleep study is ordered, it is because OSA is suspected as opposed to any of the other sleep disorders. The only dimension even the best home study devices cannot record are the various sleep stages and the duration of each. This information is not integral to an OSA diagnosis as the test otherwise provides the information necessary to evaluate and diagnose a suspected OSA case.

There are a number of credible portable home sleep test devices, but one of the most widely used is the reliable Embletta X100 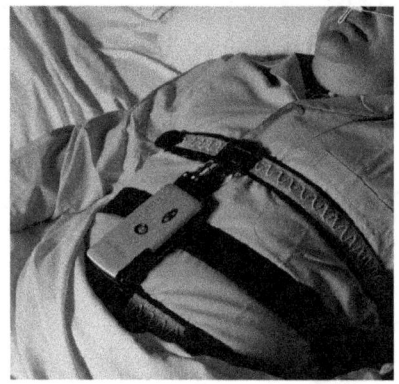 which I previously referred to. It has become the tool of preference around the globe, and especially in Europe where it has been the number one choice for home sleep tests for the last ten years or so. The Embletta X100 can only be used to diagnose OSA provided the results are confirmed by a sleep specialist. It is also most useful during the titration or adjustment period for whatever device is prescribed to treat your OSA.

Aside from the obvious convenience of the home sleep study, the unit is extremely comfortable, very accurate, and you will feel that you had a more normal sleep since you will be in your own bed.

From a health cost standpoint, it costs about five dollars to process the information collected plus whatever the sleep doctor charges to read its output and make a diagnosis. So you could be given several economical and convenient sleep studies as required to ensure that your treatment is effective in eliminating the OSA.

As far as the technical features of the Embletta X100 device, it is most acceptable to the medical profession and sleep specialists because it has a nasal cannula, pulse oximeter, and chest and abdominal straps. Some sleep specialists in sleep centers have utilized the Embletta X100 for patients who are unsuccessful with the prototypical sleep lab polysomnogram (PSG). Some patients struggle with the odor of the electrodes, suffer from claustrophobia, or cannot sleep in a strange bed with 16 electrodes attached to their body. Most patients feel that they get a more accurate sleep study done when they sleep in their own bed with the Embletta X100 device.

In fact, in Europe most of the studies prescribed *are* of the home sleep study variety due to the significant cost savings. This device has been well researched and the results correlate very accurately with the PSG done at sleep clinics.

# Chapter Seven

## Is There a Cure and What Are the Treatment Options?

The short answer to the question about whether there is a cure or not, essentially is *NO*. Having said that, it is possible that your apnea would otherwise not be present if you were a fit and lean person. There is definitely a correlation between fat mass and your ability to maintain an unobstructed upper airway. Strive for a Body Mass Index of below 18 and I can almost assure you that will positively affect you and will mitigate your OSA, although it's not quite that simple.

## The CPAP Option

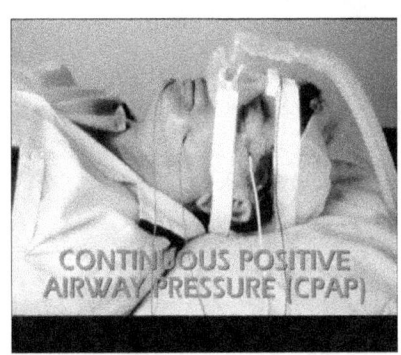

The PAP (Positive Airway Pressure) artificial ventilation system was developed in 1981 in Australia. A while later, the American Sleep Apnea Association would identify the CPAP (Continuous Positive Air Pressure) therapy as the gold standard, "go to" option to mitigate sleep apnea. Almost every doctor, every time, will recommend this treatment before anything else. They will always claim a very high success rate, although the compliance rate over an extended period of time is strikingly low. You'll likely find this out for yourself, but as the de facto gold standard you should try it out so you can make your own decision.

If you think about the number one characteristic of sleep apnea, it is recurrent pauses in breathing. A good analogy is what happens when you hold your breath (for example under water) for an extended period of time, then gasp to breathe when air is suddenly available. This is what you do when you try to sleep with an apnea. As you have read already, imagine doing this over 30 times per hour (severe sleep apnea) for 10 seconds or so each time. This is caused by the airway collapsing, so the CPAP machine is designed to pump pre-measured pressurized air into your lungs to prevent this collapse and to restore somewhat normal breathing while you try to sleep.

This artificial ventilation system is comprised of an air generator, a mask, and a hose that connects the two main components. There are different variations of the mask including one that is worn over the nose, or over the mouth, or both (a full face mask). Since the upper airway relaxes and narrows during sleep, this causes a marked drop in blood oxygen and wakes you up. The CPAP system intervenes and sends air to your lungs while preventing the air passage from collapsing during sleep.

The amount of air pressure needed to do this is determined by the sleep doctor which he bases on the severity indicated by your sleep study results. Most machines deliver 4 to 20 cm/H2O of pressurized air, and most of those diagnosed with OSA require 6 to 14 cm/H2O of pressure.

## The Three Types of CPAP Machines

Although there are three different types of CPAP equipment, they all work the same way. How they differ is in the way the pre-set pressurized air is delivered to the lungs.

The **CPAP sleep apnea machine** is the most common and the least expensive of the three. It delivers a continuous stream of air pressure to your lungs whether you are inhaling or exhaling. The continuous nature of airflow is often viewed as being problematic and a main reason for non-compliance. Although this is the original model, over the years they have become more efficient, less noisy and cumbersome, smaller and more portable.

The **Bi-level Positive Airway Pressure (BIPAP)** also known in some circles as Variable Positive Airway Pressure (VPAP) is almost the same as CPAP except for one aspect. It can deliver more pressure during inhalation and less pressure during exhalation. This offsets one of the main reasons for non-compliance with the original CPAP equipment.

The third type is the **Automatic Positive Airway Pressure (APAP)**. The working concept is the same, but this machine has the capability of auto-adjusting the air pressure on a breath by breath basis.

Obviously, the more sophisticated the equipment and the more options it has, makes for a higher price tag. Make sure you get the right machine for you, and equally important the right mask, before you invest.

## CPAP Pros and Cons in General

I am not so sure I agree, but the American Sleep Apnea Association says that using CPAP therapy is the best option for dealing with OSA. The Journal of Respiratory Therapy says that only 46% of patients are compliant after three months, and of those who continue with the therapy after this phase, 37% eventually abandon it completely. That leaves about 29 out of

100 who see it through. Even these numbers are conservative depending on where you do your research and whose data you believe. In some corners, they will claim compliancy is more like 20% after six months of use. Obviously, if this is supposed to be the medically endorsed gold standard treatment, this should be of concern to those in dire need of a successful treatment option.

There is another option, but in the meantime the issue begs many questions:

- Is CPAP truly overrated?
- Are the numerous complaints justified?
- Are earlier machines taking the rap while there are newer variants of CPAP with new options and performance improvements?
- Is the real issue a failure to choose the right mask for the individual and getting it to fit properly?

## What are the Most Common CPAP Complaints?

If CPAP is indeed the most effective treatment for OSA, it cannot be of any benefit if not used. Perhaps non-compliance statistics are a result of a lack of user knowledge and a poor job by health professionals of educating them in the first place. Nevertheless, here are the main issues.

*You are unable to adapt to the mask.* This arises because the user adjusts the headgear improperly or because the mask does not fit properly. It should fit your face snuggly to avoid air leaks, but not so tight that is feels uncomfortable or causes pain. If you have to pull it tightly to prevent leaks, it doesn't fit! Try another size or style.

*You experience nasal congestion, irritation or a runny nose.* Your nose is your airway's humidifier as it warms and moistens the air that you breathe. You will increase the production of mucus in the nose to add more moisture and this could cause congestion and a runny nose. Dryness will cause irritation, burning and sneezing, but this can be alleviated by a CPAP with a humidifier option.

*You have difficulty with nose-breathing.* Do you have allergies? See your doctor about treating them, or at least start with a good nasal spray or over-the-counter medication. Do you have sinus problems or a deviated septum? See an ear, nose and throat specialist (ENT). Try whichever style of mask you have not been using so far before you defer to more invasive or expensive alternatives.

*You experience headaches or ear pressure.* Treating OSA usually eliminates morning headache, but some people develop it while others may develop pressure or pain in their ears. It's not unlike traveling in an airplane when you have a cold as congestion can block the ear canals and changes in air pressure can cause pain when air gets trapped. They say it's best to not use CPAP when you have a cold or sinus infection, but that does nothing to mitigate your OSA. Again, try decongestants or antihistamines, but check with your doctor first.

*You remove your mask at night yet don't realize it.* Usually this is due to difficulty breathing through the nose, mask discomfort, or sleep disturbance. During an arousal you may not remember that you now wear a sleep mask, but this will likely improve over time.

*You get air in your stomach.* Occasionally you may awaken with stomach pain or gas. Ensure your head is aligned with your body or elevate your head in bed with a wedge pillow; or try tilting your mattress (or the whole bed). You can overdo this and block your airway if your head is tilted too far forward. If your doctor allows it, lowering the CPAP pressure can help, but you risk adversely affecting your treatment. Try switching to a BIPAP or APAP.

**The air is too cold.** Try a heated humidifier or try running the tubing under the covers next to your body to warm the air.

**The air is too hot.** This is harder to alter, but lower your room temperature as much as possible.

**The CPAP is too noisy.** Newer machines are quiet so this is rarely a problem. If you have an older version, get a longer tube and move the CPAP machine farther from the bed. Or, disguise the noise with a fan or other "white noise" source.

**The tubing gets in my way.** Drape the tubing behind you and over the headboard; or there is also a new option available that attaches to the bed that holds the tubing up and rotates so that it can move with you.

**You take off your mask and can't be bothered to put it back on.** When you get up at night for whatever reason, leave it on and just disconnect the tubing either at the mask or at the machine. This is easier than having to refit the mask.

**Other complaints include:**

- Mask causing skin laceration at the bridge of the nose
- Constant airflow causing dry mouth and throat
- Overall feeling of bloating
- Perception of embarrassment as the device, mask and tube make for an ugly bedside image for many
- Objection from bed partner
- Feeling of claustrophobia when wearing the mask

# What are the Positives about CPAP?

There are a few in its favor:

- Adjustable pressure for patient compliance issues.
- Most mask-related problems arise only when the mask is either too loose or too tight. There are several alternatives in terms of masks, but you must make it fit properly (which can be done).
- CPAP can be continued in conjunction with other therapy options for the treatment of sleep apnea.
- Separate attachments like humidifiers are available to offset the problem of dry mouth and throat; and antihistamines and nasal sprays can also be used to minimize side effects.
- Newer CPAP machines are made more portable and compact for ease of use during travel and for easier storage.
- Feelings of claustrophobia and anxiety can be managed with separate medication; these feelings actually have much less to do with CPAP compliance.
- Most importantly, as long as it is used CPAP unequivocally increases the level of oxygen in the blood by keeping the airway open during sleep.

# More about CPAP Variants

For those not comfortable with CPAP therapy, doctors recommend using another later version of the CPAP called the BIPAP. This unit features two variants of pressure to the lungs. For inhalation it delivers a higher amount called the Inspiratory Positive Airway Pressure (IPAP) and for exhalation it can be made to deliver slightly lower Expiratory Positive Airway Pressure (EPAP).

This machine is generally recommended for patients who suffer from neuromuscular (like ALS, more familiarly known as Lou Gehrig's Disease) and cardiopulmonary disorders over and above sleep apnea. BIPAP is more expensive than CPAP, but the side effects are more or less the same even though they are typically more tolerable. The biggest advantage of this variant is that it delivers different pressure during inhalation versus exhalation which more closely mimics normal breathing. On the downside, the amounts of titrated pressure need constant monitoring.

I am personally biased towards an oral device, but if you can remain unbiased you might find the positives outweigh the negatives. I would think too about combining an oral device with using a CPAP. Discontinuation of CPAP is a matter of personal choice, but is a bad idea and a death wish if you do not replace it with another form of treatment.

# More about Different Masks

A range of CPAP masks are available. Some feature full face masks that cover your mouth and nose, with straps that stretch across your forehead and cheeks. These may make some people feel claustrophobic, but they work well at providing a stable fit if you move around a lot in your sleep. Other masks feature nasal pillows that fit under your nose and straps that cover less of your face. These can feel more acceptable and could work better if you wear glasses or read with the mask on. Some nasal pillow systems obstruct vision much less than do full face masks, yet they may not work if you move around a lot or sleep on your side.

Pay attention to size because most masks come in different sizes. Just because you're a certain size in one type of mask doesn't mean you'll be the same size in another type. CPAP masks are usually adjustable, but have an expert (doctor or supplier) to show you how to adjust your mask to get the best fit. Manufacturer product instructions also can help show you how to do this.

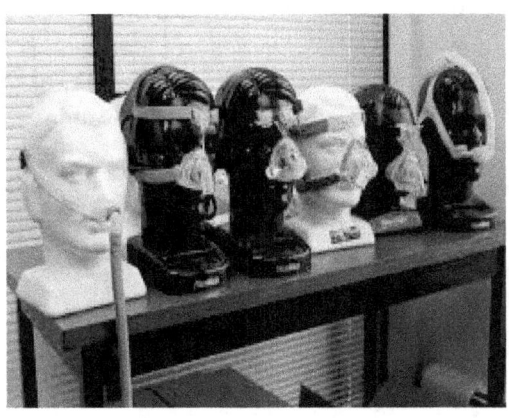

Get used to wearing the mask first. For example, start by practicing wearing just the mask for short periods of time while you're awake like while watching TV. Then try wearing the mask and hose with the air pressure on during the daytime while you're awake. Once you become accustomed to how that feels, take a nap and/or sleep with it every time (night and during day naps). Inconsistently wearing the CPAP device may delay getting used to it. Stick with it for several weeks or more to see if the mask and pressure settings you have will work for you.

If you have difficulty tolerating forced air, you may be able to overcome this by using a "ramp" feature on a fully optioned machine. Ramping allows you to start with low air pressure, followed by an automatic, gradual increase in the pressure to your prescribed setting as you fall asleep. The ramping rate needs to be adjusted by your doctor.

One final thing that may help out if you go the CPAP route is a pillow that makes it easier to sleep with the unit. You can try a CPAP and Mask pillow by clicking the link.

## The Oral Appliance Option

While CPAP is the first choice of doctors treating sleep apnea, it's not necessarily the first choice of those diagnosed with sleep apnea who are in search of a treatment and who are aware there is a oral (dental) solution available. Therein lies the real issue. In the introduction to this book I mentioned the hundreds of books, white papers and websites focused on snoring and sleep apnea, yet only a very few of them even discuss this option. A huge number of doctors whose specialty is sleep medicine can hardly believe a patient would even consider a dental solution viable. When compared to the medical community's gold standard CPAP option, widespread patient rejection of the gold standard therapy has sent actual usage statistics plummeting as rates of non-compliance soar.

If you fall into this category, The American Academy of Sleep Medicine recommends the use of a dental appliance for sleep apnea patients as a totally viable option for treating mild to moderate sleep apnea; and for those who simply cannot tolerate or otherwise remain compliant with traditional CPAP therapy.

*Who should NOT use an oral (dental) appliance?* If you have a temporomandibular joint (TMJ) disorder, pain in the oral and/or facial region, have either loose, damaged or no teeth, an oral solution may not work for you immediately. You should get the TMJ problem fixed first, or otherwise tend to the facial pain before exploring an oral device for snoring and sleep apnea. In terms of problems with the teeth themselves, you can understand that the device needs to anchor itself to your teeth. So it is a prerequisite they be in reasonable shape in order for the patient to expect success.

## How does a Mandibular Advancement Device (MAD) work?

Though some doctors may recommend the use of a dental device (approved by the FDA) to manage mild to moderate OSA, in many cases this device is totally effective in mitigating *severe* OSA as well. My apnea is severe at 59 AHI and my device brought this down to 6 AHI in a subsequent sleep test. Don't let a doctor dictate whether or not you choose this option if you have severe OSA. You won't know its effectiveness until you try it.

This type of device is worn in the mouth during sleep. They are user-friendly, safe and unobtrusive, but only a dentist trained in sleep therapy should be used to select, customize and fit the device. The purpose of an oral device is to allow you to breathe normally and without any pauses interrupting sleep. This can be achieved only when the airway is open allowing for the free passage of air. This results by bringing the lower jaw forward, which in turn keeps the upper respiratory muscles tightened.

It will also have a positive impact on snoring as vibration of the airway tissue is significantly reduced. It also keeps the tongue from dropping back and blocking the airway since your tongue is anatomically attached to the inside of the jaw. The best way to think of it is, the device simply keeps your upper and lower jaw aligned at night while sleeping the same way it is during the daytime.

## What are the Types of Oral Appliances?

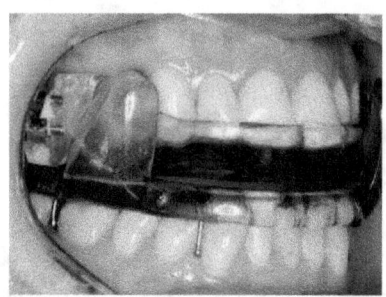

Modern appliances allow users to speak, drink, or yawn with the device in place. Basically, there are two types of dental appliances recommended for sleep apnea patients. Both of these work to achieve the primary aim of the therapy – to keep airways open. They are the Mandibular Advancement Device (MAD) and the Tongue Retaining Device (TRD).

The **Mandibular Advancement Device** is the most used and looks very much like a typical sports mouth guard used by athletes. It works by advancing the lower jaw. Because the tongue is also linked to the jaw, the advancing action keeps the tongue out of the way and prevents it from causing an obstruction in air flow.

Most oral appliances are not 100% effective when they are first inserted. The uvula and soft palate tissues can be quite swollen due to snoring and/or smoking. As the swelling subsides, the appliance is slowly adjusted to move the mandible and tongue further forward, sometimes a month or two of titration which you can do yourself. During the titration period, it is often advisable to test the efficacy of the oral appliance with a home sleep study that your dentist can arrange for you (for example by using the Embletta X100).

The **Tongue Retaining Device** works by placing the tongue in a forward position in the mouth to prevent it from receding backwards and obstructing breathing. This device also advances the jaw to assist in the effort to keep the tongue forward. The device has a suction bulb which is needed to hold the tongue tip to the teeth and lips to keep it in place. Some versions of the more popular oral devices can be modified to both advance the mandible *and* keep the tongue forward.

## What are the Pros & Cons of Dental Appliances?

Depending on your condition and the cause of your sleep apnea, the sleep therapy trained dentist will tell you what type of dental appliance would best suit you. As mentioned, medical doctors are divided on the use of dental appliances. Some believe they worsen symptoms, but that is usually only when not properly built for you and not subsequently adjusted (titrated) for you. Success is contingent on proper treatment, user tolerance factors, and expectations from the therapy.

*Benefits of Dental Appliances can Include:*

- Significant reduction of severity of symptoms
- Significant reduction of snoring
- Much more user-friendly than CPAP
- Much higher compliance due to convenience of use, size, usability and maintenance
- Significant improvement in quality and quantity of sleep.
- Better value as treatment cost is lower than CPAP

*Potential Negative Aspects of Dental Appliances may Affect:*

- Intimacy with your partner
- Increased production of saliva
- Gum irritation
- Might be less effective if you're a side sleeper
- Might not be as effective as CPAP (but higher compliance)
- MAD therapy may not be reimbursable by insurance
- Might experience dry mouth and lips, sore tongue, sore jaw, oral pain and discomfort (until used to device)
- Might cause damage to teeth and jaw over long term

Oral appliances only work if your sleep apnea is caused by your jaw or tongue obstructing your airway. Similarly, the TRD will be ineffective if the cause of your sleep apnea is NOT your tongue.

If you are CPAP intolerant, this is a legitimate alternative. A 2005 clinical study conducted by American Academy of Sleep Medicine found that the dental appliance for sleep apnea is a most worthy treatment option for OSA, particularly for those who are CPAP intolerant or who want to avoid surgery. It is also the ideal treatment for those who drive for a living due to its simplicity and convenience.

# Surgical Option Overview

While OSA is indeed a serious issue, so is a surgical solution. My recommendation is to NOT go down this road unless it is the only chance of successfully treating your apnea. I speak from personal experience. Your polysomnogram will indicate if this option is in play and will call for a further physical examination by an ENT specialist (hopefully one who is also trained in sleep medicine - if not get a second opinion). Depending on the objective, most surgeries remove excess tissue from different sites in the upper airway tract so that you can breathe without pause. Some doctors may characterize it as reconstruction of the soft tissue of the uvula or palate. In considering surgery, one criterion is what is called the Mallampati Score. There are four grades, and the higher the grade - the smaller the air passage.

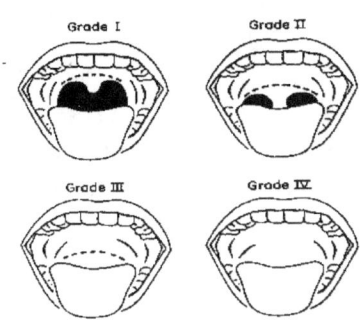

Grade I    Grade II

Grade III    Grade IV

Sometimes surgery is called for when a patient refuses to remain compliant with CPAP and creates a critically deteriorating health condition. Other times surgery is for purposes of fixing snoring, but also positions the patient for subsequent CPAP or oral appliance treatment therapies for OSA. The medical community will tell you that surgery success rates are only in the area of 50-65% and may have no positive effect on your problem other than it might reduce the AHI count slightly. Like any surgery, it could even make the condition worse. Here are the usual procedures:

***Uvulopalatopharyngoplasty (UPPP)*** removes soft tissue on the back of the throat including all or part of the uvula (the soft flap of tissue that hangs down at the back of the mouth) and parts of the soft palate and the throat tissue behind it. If tonsils and adenoids are present, they are removed and you'll probably still need CPAP. A UPPP is painful, takes weeks to recover from it, can cause excess mucous, changes in voice, swallowing issues, regurgitation of fluids through the nose or mouth, impaired sense of smell, recurrence of apnea, and can make CPAP ineffective later. Don't do it unless you're going to die otherwise.

***Laser-Assisted Uvulopalatoplasty (LAUP)*** is a variation of a UPPP. I had it done 22 years ago for snoring. Don't do it either, for all the same reasons. It removes less tissue at the back of the throat 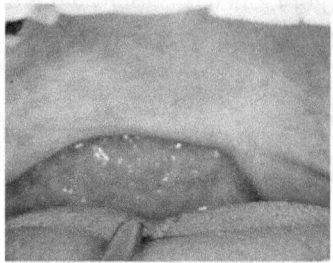 than a UPPP and can be done in a doctor's office. The doctor I had did not even mention the words "sleep apnea." It was painful, did not work, and today I have no uvula (see the image). I am certain that when I eventually die, it will be because of inhaling crumbs or some other residual food left on my tongue that I vacuum straight into my windpipe. I regret ever having this done. Don't do it unless there is no option!

A ***Pillar Palatal Implant*** is a better alternative to either of the above surgeries. It is a non-invasive surgical treatment for mild-to-moderate sleep apnea and snoring in particular. A doctor inserts three short pieces of polyester string into the soft palate. It can be done in his office in about 10 minutes under local anesthesia. Studies reveal it works as well as UPPP with less pain and quicker recovery time. Watch a three minute video that explains the procedure. Just click here, or go to your browser and type http://www.pillarprocedure.com/what-is-it/index.htm

A ***Tracheostomy*** *(or tracheotomy)* used to be the only treatment for sleep apnea. It is simple inasmuch as the surgeon makes an opening through the neck into the windpipe and inserts a tube. It is almost 100% successful, but it requires a quarter-sized opening in the throat. This often leaves you with medical and psychological problems associated with recovery. Today it is rarely performed unless your sleep apnea is life threatening.

***Other Procedures*** to correct facial abnormalities or obstructions that cause sleep apnea may be used alone or combined with each other, or with a UPPP. Most are invasive and reserved for those with severe sleep apnea who previously failed to respond to or comply with CPAP, and they include:

- **Hyoid Advancement** - bone under the chin is moved forward, pulling the tongue muscle along with it

- **Maxillary** advancement (MMA), which moves the upper (maxilla) or lower (mandible) jawbone forward

- **Nasal Obstruction** (deviated septum) that contribute to snoring and other symptoms (I had this done too)

- **Genioglossus** - tongue advancement

- **Temperature Controlled Radio Frequency Ablation** - tongue reduction

# Diets Don't Work but Losing Fat Does

*This is not a diet book you're reading*, but I will refer you to a book called **The Gabriel Method.** In it, the author Jon Gabriel talks about the nine hidden fat triggers that got you into this condition in the first place, and as a sedentary truck or bus driver he will tell you how to shut them off. It is not what you think, but the ninth trigger itself is sleep apnea. Here is what he says:

> *People say sleeping too much makes you fat, but the opposite can also be true. Sleep apnea is a disorder that causes you to stop breathing as you sleep, sometimes hundreds of times a night, without even realizing it. The result is shallow, interrupted sleep – and weight gain.*
>
> *Sleep apnea reduces your blood oxygen to dangerously low levels, so **your body is starving for oxygen**. You then become chronically exhausted, which gives you junk food cravings. It also makes you*

*more irritable, releases cortisol into your system, and makes you prone to negative emotions – another Fat Trigger.*

*Lack of sleep also influences the levels of leptin and ghrelin hormones in your body, which control feelings of hunger and fullness. "When you don't get enough sleep, it drives leptin levels down, which means you don't feel as satisfied after you eat," explains Michael Breus, PhD, Director of The Sleep Disorders Center in Atlanta.*

Here's what I say. There is a significant and intertwined relationship between your sleep habits and your metabolism. Everybody knows that around age 40 we all tend to add pounds to some degree, but if you suffer from sleep deprivation you are probably expediting and exacerbating that process. It's a real 'chicken and egg' scenario since sleep apnea also seems to become more prevalent at the same age.

Read The Gabriel Method to understand the psychology involved, then aside from getting proper sleep there is not much you have to do differently about fat other than focusing on what you consume (diet) and how active you are (exercise). As we know, a lifestyle on the road sets you up to fail in these areas unless you are really focused on improving your health as it relates to breathing during sleep. Later on go to the website at 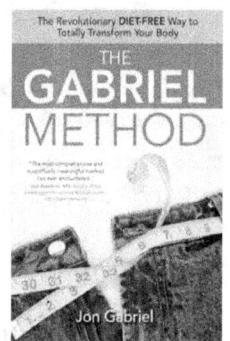 http://www.thegabrielmethod.com/store, and once inside, click on the tab called ***FREE Stuff***.

With your upper airway collapsing over and over again while trying to sleep, your blood oxygen level starts to bottom out. Your brain recognizes this and wakes you up. In the process, sleep is disrupted and does not refresh you. Obesity sets in along with increasing carbon dioxide levels, which is created by metabolism within your body. Since carbon dioxide is removed by your lungs, you're not going to get rid of it if you are not breathing properly. These higher levels will cause drowsiness and at worst, unconsciousness, coma, and then death.

Now with metabolism messed up, the resulting excessive daytime sleepiness can affect food choices thus increasing caloric intake, including caffeine-containing products. Along with that, you'll be less motivated to exercise because it's harder to do on the road anyhow. You have to understand this and get off this cycle. It is hard for a driver, but you have to figure out how to get it done.

1. Eliminate junk food like soda pop, candy, and fast food.
2. Eat more fruits, vegetables, and whole grains.
3. Cut portion sizes.
4. Drink as much water as you can consume.
5. Get 30-60 minutes of exercise daily doing anything, including simply walking (you're only driving 10 hours or so a day, figure out how you're going to get it done).

Pay attention to food labels. Stop drinking juices and soda pop. Drink more water. Cut out manufactured foods high in sugar. Avoid fast food.

Do simple stretching, walking, or swimming where you can. It is going to be tough, but the alternative is you're not going to get past the sleep apnea so you will get sicker and sicker and become unable to beat the resulting health issues.

## Other Devices - Pros and Cons

Let me be clear about the various products you can buy to deal with sleep issues; whether you self-diagnose or get a formal diagnosis of having a sleep apnea, if you're like most people you will likely try all sorts of shortcuts in order to mitigate your symptoms. Your sleep apnea treatment options are CPAP, Oral Device, Surgery, and losing lots of fat. That's it, that's all for now. Everything else you encounter will primarily be designed to help you stop snoring. Having said that, while not a treatment for sleep apnea, anything you do have success with, will give you marginally better sleep quality but you will not fix an apnea.

- There are pillows designed to properly align your head and neck to keep your airway open as throat muscles relax during sleep

- There are all sorts of throat and nasal sprays that will claim to stop snoring (although I'm not sure how)

- There are nasal strips designed to keep your nostrils wide open to allow more air intake

- There are chin straps designed to keep your mandible aligned thus keeping the airway open (not much help if you can't get enough air to breathe causing you to wake)

- There are sleep positioning devices to keep you on your side and off your back while sleeping (think of the t-shirt with tennis balls sewn into the back)

- There are acupressure and reflex therapy devices based on eastern medicine for sale everywhere

- There are biofeedback machines that sense you are snoring and give you a mild shock to cause you to reposition yourself

Some or all of these devices may cause some improvement in the quality of sleep, but they will not treat your apnea. I will list sources for these products in the next chapter on support if you

want to investigate them, but a few things that you could try that will pay some dividends are these:

## *Tilted Bed*

There is really no downside to trying to sleep on a tilted bed where the headboard end is about eight inches higher than the footboard end. In this situation, gravity has a lessened effect on the physics of the throat and there is a lessened propensity for the mandible (lower jaw) to recede and close off the airway. Breathing is somewhat easier since there is less pressure on the diaphragm and snoring is reduced.

Additionally, there is less pooling of blood in the upper half of the body which has the effect of lowering blood pressure and mitigating potential for congestive heart failure. The other benefit is that it helps mitigate acid reflux often brought on by that truck stop diet. Perhaps try a wedge pillow that may accomplish the same thing. You can check out the Science of Sleep Wedge device I use by clicking the name.

## *Sleep Positioning Device*

Learn how to sleep on your side and it will mitigate (to a certain extent) your mandible receding and blocking your airway. Most people can't help rolling over on their back during the night so these positioning devices are designed to make sleeping on your back uncomfortable so you'll roll back over onto your side.

You can purchase a device that does this for you, or the homemade method is to put a tennis ball inside of a sock and then pin the sock to the back of your shirt. It's an effective way of preventing you from sleeping on your back. The Zzoma product (pictured) is a belt with foam rubber positioners in the back that you wear to bed to make it difficult to roll onto your back. The Rematee product uses similar foam rubber positioning devices.

The Therapeutic Pillow Side Sleeper works differently. It's a device designed to fit between the legs encouraging your body to lie comfortably on its side. Note that they also offer a Body Wedge Aligner if additional support is desired. Do your own research by going to:

- Zzoma (www.zzomasleep.com)

- Rematee (www.antisnoreshirt.com)

- Therapeutic Pillow Side Sleeper (http://www.the-pillow.com.au/general/category_snoring.php)

## *Oral Devices Not Provided by a Dentist*

There are only two circumstances where I would recommend this option. Firstly, if you will otherwise do nothing about getting tested, or otherwise do nothing to try and deal with your sleep situation; and secondly, so you can see for yourself if an oral device concept is likely to help you mitigate the negative circumstances created by your sleep disorder.

There are a couple of oral devices that cost around $60 that you can test for 30 days for the $10 cost of shipping it to you. They are not custom designed and they only last 9 to 12 months at best. What they will do though is give you an idea if an dentist prescribed oral device will be a good option to invest in later on.

There are a few *caveats* that you should be aware of. By reducing or eliminating snoring before you have a sleep study, you may be masking a warning that sleep apnea may be a problem for you. Second, because these appliances *do* hold the jaw in a forward position, there are problems occasionally like shifting of tooth position and pain in the joints to contend with. Finally, these appliances may *not* function effectively and lead you to believe (erroneously) that oral appliances are not worthy.

The chart below is not complete, but seems to include the most popular over-the-counter devices:

| | SnoreMender | SnoreRx | Ripsnore | PureSleep |
|---|---|---|---|---|
| **Money Back Guarantee** | *90 days* | *30 days* | *45 days* | *30 days* |
| **Works Without Fitting** | *Yes* | *No* | *No* | *No* |
| **# of Fitting Attempts** | *Not required* | | *5 then needs replacing* | *3-4 then needs replacing* |
| **Hinged to Let Mouth Move Naturally** | *Yes* | *No, jaw locked in place* | *No, jaw locked in place* | *No, jaw locked in place* |
| **Stays in Place if Mouth Open** | *Yes* | *No* | *Yes* | *No* |
| **Allows Mouth Breathing** | *Yes* | *Only through 2 small holes* | *Only through 2 small holes* | *Restricted* |
| **Side to Side Jaw Movement** | *Yes* | *No* | *No* | *No* |
| **Flexible Frame for Comfort** | *Yes* | *No* | *No* | *No* |
| **Ease of Cleaning** | *Easy shape, hand wash with soap* | *Awkward gaps to clean* | *Awkward gaps to clean* | *Awkward gaps to clean & needs cleaning solutions* |
| **Product Lifetime** | *Average of 9-18 months* | | *Average of 6-18 months* | *Average of 6-12 months* |

If you have successfully tried out one of these do-it-yourself boil-and-bite appliances and have found it to be successful, you owe it to yourself to experience the real deal and effectiveness of a professionally made appliance. Beware, these Internet devices may be uncomfortable, bulky and may keep falling out; and be clear - they cannot compete with a professionally made device.

Most dentists will endorse a legitimate non-custom oral appliance you can try for purposes of kicking the tires on the mandibular advancement device (MAD) concept. None are comparable in their construction, quality and effectiveness to one that a dentist will prescribe and have custom made for you, but it will help you test drive the concept. My research seems to reveal that when a dentist recommends an over the counter device, they tend to mention the PureSleep device first. To save time, you can either click here or go to http://www.trypuresleep.com and have a look.

Remember, most are sold for purposes of stopping snoring, not mitigating sleep apnea. Stay focused on getting this done right. You can tell whose chart that was, but the comparison may help if you choose to try one out.

Here's a few others if you want to check them out:

- Snore Guard (www.somni.com)
- ZQuiet (www.zquiet.com)
- SnoreMeds (www.snoremeds.com)
- SnoreMate (www.snoremate.net)

## What To Do About Your Suspected OSA in the Meantime?

To start with, forget about energy drinks except in an emergency. They will keep you awake for awhile, but taking in too many caffeinated drinks is not a good solution to driver fatigue. Your fatigue is caused by sleep deprivation so don't think these drinks will fix that. Your sleep deprivation has been caused by a number of factors already discussed, but the real cause is an irregular sleep pattern and an inability to adjust. We humans are not like racoons or skunks, we weren't designed to be nocturnal. But driving schedules for truckers and bus drivers (in the case of this book) are a fact of that work lifestyle. You would think some of us could adapt, but we never really do.

To review, the NTSB says that almost 20% of all fatal crashes (involving large trucks) are caused by driver fatigue, plus 7% of all accidents period (fatal or non-fatal). The early hours of the morning and just after lunch time are the peak times for fatigue related accidents. Although few admit it, some drivers falsify HOS reports so they can keep driving and make their deadlines. And although they too will never admit it, some companies turn a blind eye while hoping nothing bad comes of it.

Having said that, everybody from regulatory bodies to transportation companies are tightening the thumbscrews on drivers, so just be proactive and get with the program first.

Now that you've decided to deal with your own issues by getting tested and treated as predicated by your diagnosis, here is what to do in the meantime (and even after beginning treatment):

1: GET ENOUGH SLEEP BEFORE GETTING BEHIND THE WHEEL. *Shoot for between seven and eight hours. Where possible, avoid driving while your body is naturally drowsy (12AM to 6AM and 2PM to 4PM).*

2: MAINTAIN A HEALTHY DIET. *Skipping meals or eating at irregular hours leads to fatigue. Both going to sleep with an empty stomach or right after a heavy meal can interfere with sleep. Try a light snack just before sleep.*

3: POWER NAP. *They should last 10 to 45 minutes - then allow at least 15 minutes after waking to fully recover before starting to drive.*

4: AVOID TAKING MEDICATIONS THAT MAY INDUCE DROWSINESS JUST BEFORE DRIVING. *Common medicines include tranquilizers, sleeping pills, allergy medicines and cold medicines.*

5: RECOGNIZE THE SIGNALS AND DANGERS OF DROWSINESS. *Pay attention to frequent yawning, heavy eyes, and blurred vision. Also, smoking, turning up the radio, drinking coffee, opening the window, and energy drinks are not cures and may give you a false sense of security.*

# My Personal Recommendation

It's not complicated. You already know if you're a candidate for sleep apnea. You are now aware, not only of the risks involved in driving for a living anyway, but how you compound those risks while driving with sleep apnea. You are also now aware of the associated medical risks attached to sleep apnea, even if you do *not* drive for a living.

You should have a comfort level with the fact that you will not compromise your license provided you seek a diagnosis, receive treatment, and remain compliant. You are aware that testing, where not currently in effect, *will become* a condition of employment. Even owner-operators won't escape testing because their Department of Transport issued license will also soon be issued on the basis of satisfactorily passing a sleep test.

Take the initiative now and complete the self-diagnosis steps I provided for you. Take the results to your doctor for review. Give this book to your relatives and to your dentist; or tell them where they can get their own copy. If your dentist is not already qualified to provide treatment, encourage him/her to take steps to do so because close to 30% of his existing patients will likely have sleep apnea and he/she can help them.

As you've read, there is a wide variety of non-surgical devices and techniques which are all different. Some will help more than others depending on your lifestyle and sleeping habits. You may want to try one or two strategies (even two at the same time), but remember that the only effective and current treatments for sleep apnea are the CPAP, a 'designed for you' oral appliance, surgery, and one more new and innovative option I will elaborate on in chapter nine.

# Chapter Eight

## Sleep Medicine - Sleep Therapy

For something that has occupied about one-third of the life of every human that has ever lived, it is surprising that sleep is a relatively new specialty. It has only been since the middle of the 20th century that research has provided increasing knowledge and answered many questions about sleep-wake functioning. While it is *now* a rapidly evolving field, there is still a drastic shortage of doctors trained as experts when measured against the prevalence of sleep disorders.

Dental sleep medicine also now qualifies for board certification in many countries. In some of those same countries, the sleep researchers and the doctors who treat patients may be the same people. The first sleep clinics in the United States were just recently established in the 1970s by interested doctors and technicians with the study, diagnosis and treatment of obstructive sleep apnea being their first priority. As late as 1999, virtually any American doctor, with no specific training in sleep medicine could hang a shingle, open a sleep lab and call himself a specialist.

Regarding the incentive for this book, the US National Transportation Safety Board has discovered that the leading cause of fatal-to-the-driver heavy truck crashes is fatigue related at 31%, with alcohol and other drug use at 29%.

Competence in sleep medicine requires an understanding of very diverse disorders, many with similar symptoms like excessive daytime sleepiness, where in the absence of sleep deprivation there is almost always an identifiable cause and treatable sleep disorder like sleep apnea.

Since sleep apnea was first described in medical literature in 1965, the medical importance of sleep was recognized. The medical community began paying more attention than previously to primary sleep disorders such as sleep apnea as well as the role and quality of sleep in other conditions. By the 1970s and within the next 20 years, clinics and laboratories devoted to the study of sleep and the treatment of its disorders had been founded with most sleep doctors primarily concerned with apnea. However, to that point there was nothing to restrict the use of the title "sleep doctor," so a need for standards arose.

Basic medical training has paid little attention to sleep problems. A survey in 1990–91 of 37 American medical schools revealed at the time that sleep and sleep disorders were "covered" in less than two (2) hours of total teaching time on average. A 2002 survey of more than 500 primary care doctors reported their knowledge of sleep disorders as:

*Excellent – 0%   Good – 10%   Fair – 60%   Poor – 30%*

A review of more than 50 studies indicated that both doctors and patients are reluctant to discuss sleep complaints because of the perception that treatments are ineffective or associated with risks; and physicians may have avoided dealing with sleep issues because it was taking more than the normal allotted time for receiving patients for other matters.

Enter the dentist. He is not qualified to medically diagnose, but he's *rapidly* becoming an equal player in sleep therapy treatment. I stated earlier that dental devices are perceived to be effective for mild to moderate sleep apnea, but I'm here to tell you that it took my severe apnea from 59 AHI to 6 AHI. I can also tell you that compliance is near 90% (I am 100% compliant unless I fall asleep watching TV or reading, which I seldom do now).

## Who You Should Share This Book With

To share the book is to share the information it contains. Having read this far, you already know more than what 95% of the population knows about sleep apnea, its dangers, and potential for negatively impacting lives. In particular, you now really understand the ramifications of operating a vehicle (commercial or otherwise) if you have a sleep disorder along with the associated risks for yourself and those you share the road with.

To start, you will inherently know people who will benefit from this knowledge. Share this book or tell your family, relatives and friends where to get it and why they need it. Do the same with others who also drive to earn a living.

I would be willing to bet that your personal doctor is not much more than casually knowledgeable about this information. As of this writing, there is nowhere near enough medical doctors who have made it their specialty to deal with sleep disorders and the prevalence this affliction is taking on. The onus is on doctors to catch up and learn as much as possible in order to properly guide their existing patients when they suspect a sleep disorder may be at the root of much of what ails their patient. Show your doctor what you've been reading.

There is less onus on your dentist, but more upside to their existing practice if they become knowledgeable and interested in adding sleep therapy to their treatment menu. Show your dentist the book, or tell him/her about it and where you got it. My personal opinion is that the dentist has an even greater potential for helping people improve the quality of their lives because he can be much more proactive with his existing clientele, as opposed to a medical doctor who inherently is more reactive. You go to your MD when you're sick, but you visit the dentist on a much more regular basis if you're actually taking care of your teeth.

## The Dentist's Role in Sleep Apnea Treatment

**Dental Sleep Medicine** is an area of a dental practice that focuses on the management of sleep-related breathing disorders including snoring and obstructive sleep apnea through the use of oral appliance therapy, and potentially upper airway surgery (through his diligence and referrals to an E.N.T. specialist).

Patients visit their dentist more often than any other health care professional. Therefore, dentists have an excellent opportunity to help educate, participate in the diagnosis, and treat their patients with oral appliances when it is determined to be the treatment of choice.

Dentists together with sleep physicians are challenged to respond to the health risks and economic impact of untreated sleep apnea and excessive daytime sleepiness. This partnership tasks physicians with the recognition and diagnosis of sleep disorders, while dentists provide an alternative treatment option.

Dentists have pioneered the use of oral appliance therapy for the treatment of sleep apnea and sleep related breathing disorders. To revisit, an oral appliance is simply a device worn in the mouth only during sleep. The device fits like a sports mouth guard or orthodontic retainer and prevents the airway from collapsing by either holding the tongue or supporting the jaw in a forward position. With an oral appliance, dentists can minimize or eliminate the symptoms of sleep apnea in mild to moderate (and some severe) cases.

A physician is responsible for the diagnosis of sleep disorders and for recommending a treatment. A board certified sleep medicine physician at an accredited sleep center uses an overnight sleep study to detect and diagnose sleep apnea. Once a patient is diagnosed with sleep apnea or a sleep related breathing disorder, a dental sleep specialist may then provide treatment. A dentist assists patients in the selection and fitting of an oral appliance and provides long-term follow-up care.

A dental sleep specialist may recommend upper airway surgery when other treatment options are unsuccessful in eliminating the symptoms of sleep apnea, or when they are not tolerated by patients. To assist practitioners in the diagnosis of OSA, the focus is on three areas as relates to airway obstruction: *Nasal (your nose), Oropharyngeal (your mouth) and Hypopharyngeal (your throat).*

**Nasal Obstructions:** Prior to treatment, the sleep trained dentist must determine whether or not there are any nasal obstructions that would interfere with the patient's ability to breathe through their nose. If the patient is a chronic mouth breather, the dentist will refer the patient an E.N.T. specialist to check for a deviated septum, enlarged turbinates, polyps or other nasal obstructions. A determination must be made whether or not the nasal mucosa is swollen due to allergies which might cause a nasal obstruction.

A diagnostic device known as a *Rhinometer* is an initial screening device used to determine if there is a nasal obstruction in either nostril. The rhinometer is an accurate, non-invasive device which evaluates the potential obstruction by sending sound waves up the nose and any obstructions are recorded on a computer. This evaluation of the nasal cavity is also important if the sleep specialist decides to use the CPAP device to force air through the nose.

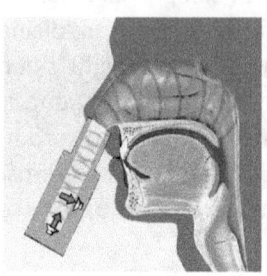

Obviously, if there is a nasal obstruction, the pressure would have to be much higher on the CPAP device. Compliance with CPAP treatment is higher when the pressure is lower. Therefore, an evaluation of a patient's nasal airway is an important prerequisite to a successful oral appliance or CPAP therapy.

**Oropharyngeal Obstructions:** Prior to the fabrication of the oral appliance or CPAP therapy, an evaluation must be done of the oral cavity to check for obstructions. The areas of concern would be enlarged tonsils or adenoids, large tongue, enlarged uvula, large mandibular tori (excess bone that grows on the mandible inside your mouth), excess tissue in the area of the soft palate, or enlarged torus palatines (excess bone growth on the palate). Patients with narrow maxillary arches and high palates are also more susceptible to snoring and OSA. Oropharyngeal obstructions must be surgically corrected prior to oral appliance or CPAP therapy.

**Hypopharyngeal Obstructions:** Oral appliances are most effective when there are no nasal or oropharyngeal obstructions and the problem is behind the tongue in the area of the throat. Class II skeletal patients with retrognathic mandibles are the patients that are more likely to have hypopharyngeal obstructions. Their lower jaws already recede, which subsequently causes their tongues to recede. This is particularly serious when the patient sleeps on their back so the tongue falls even further back and blocks the airway. If the tongue partially blocks the airway, the patient snores. If it completely blocks the airway for 10 seconds or more, for more than 6 times an hour, the patient is diagnosed with OSA. The main function of the oral appliance is to move the lower jaw forward, increase the vertical space and subsequently move the tongue forward to open up the pharyngeal airway.

A **Pharyngometer** is a diagnostic device utilized to diagnose the size of the airway. It is utilized at the initial appointment to check

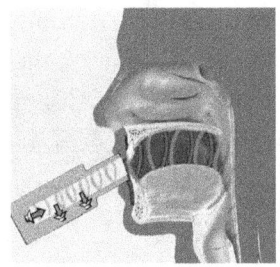

the patient's normal daytime airway and the collapsed airway at night. To assess the size of the collapsed airway at night, the patient is instructed to exhale all the air from their lungs and a measurement of the airway is taken. The normal size of a collapsed airway is two centimetres. Patients with OSA usually have a much smaller collapsed airway. Bite registrations in different positions are taken to try and see how large the airway may be increased. By moving the mandible forward at different vertical heights, you can determine if the oral appliance will open the airway in that position significantly. In most cases, when a bite registration

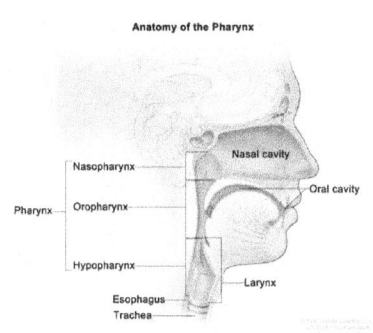

Anatomy of the Pharynx

reveals that the airway opens significantly, and when the oral appliance is fabricated in that position, the treatment is usually successful.

The results using different bite registrations are not always successful if the patient has a physiologically narrow airway or has excessive swelling in the area of the uvula and soft palate due to excessive snoring or smoking. The pharyngometer helps to give the dentist a starting position to fabricate the oral appliance. It is important to select a position that is comfortable for the patient. It is advisable then to use an oral appliance that can be adjusted to move the mandible slowly forward to reduce the snoring and OSA.

As mentioned previously, airway obstructions in the nasal and oropharyngeal (mouth) areas must be eliminated prior to the fabrication of the oral appliance. When oral appliances are utilized in these cases, they are highly effective. The success rate with oral appliance therapy is over 90%. If you cannot properly diagnose the problem, treatment will be less successful.

Patients much prefer to wear an oral appliance rather than the CPAP device. However, for severe OSA, the CPAP is still the first treatment of choice. If a patient is unable to wear the CPAP and they have severe OSA, or if they have mild to moderate OSA, the oral appliance becomes the treatment of choice.

If a dentist incorporates sleep therapy into their existing practice, he will start helping these patients achieve a higher level of overall health and extend their lifespan. In Canada, most insurance companies will pay for the CPAP device but will not pay for oral appliances. In the USA, many medical plans now pay for both CPAP and oral appliances. Jurisdictions who are not getting on board with this concept, are not really saving money. They miss the fact that they are actually paying out these dollars anyhow, but for all of the other medical complications caused by the apnea. It is a very narrow view of reality, but I feel that one day they will figure it all out.

It is the responsibility of both the medical and dental professions to identify patients who have airway obstructions leading to snoring and sleep apnea. It is also advisable to have a bed partner participate in the initial evaluation as relates to the patient's sleep habits and daytime sleepiness as it will normally be extremely accurate.

All dentists should be encouraged to give the Epworth Sleepiness Test to all of their all patients who snore, as snoring is one of the main symptoms of obstructive sleep apnea. They should also educate their staff, including receptionists, dental assistants and hygienists regarding the diagnosis and treatment of these patients. Hygienists are particularly important in conveying the information to patients and asking them to complete the Epworth Sleepiness Scale.

For any patient that has an Epworth Sleepiness Scale result higher than eight (8), it is recommended they seek medical attention in terms of a sleep study in order to diagnose the presence (or absence) of OSA. Patients who snore but do *not* have OSA may still be treated by the dentist with an oral appliance. Prior to the fabrication of the oral appliance, the dentist must receive a report from a sleep specialist stating that the patient actually does *not* have sleep apnea. When the patient only snores and does *not* have sleep apnea, no follow-up sleep study is necessary. If the patient *is* diagnosed with mild to moderate OSA and the sleep specialist and patient agree, the dentist can then fabricate an oral appliance.

After the oral appliance has been adjusted over several months, the patient must have a follow-up sleep study (PSG) to confirm the efficacy of the appliance. It is imperative that the dentist establish a good working relationship with a sleep specialist in the sleep lab if they want to be successful in the field of sleep dentistry.

Most sleep specialists will welcome the opportunity to work with competent dentists. Once a good relationship has been established, this will result in referrals for patients with mild sleep apnea and those who cannot tolerate their CPAP device.

As described in an earlier chapter, another excellent diagnostic device is the Embletta X100, a home sleep study device. Patients much prefer this home sleep study compared to the hospital sleep study (polysomnogram). The Embletta X100 cannot be used to diagnose OSA unless the results are interpreted by a sleep specialist, but the device is always useful during the titration or adjustment period for an oral appliance. Most oral appliances are not 100% effective when they are first inserted. The uvula and soft palate tissues can be quite swollen due to snoring and/or smoking. As the swelling subsides, the appliance is slowly adjusted to move the mandible and tongue further forward, sometimes taking a couple of months.

During the titration period, it is advisable to test the efficacy of the oral appliance with the home sleep study. The advantage of this device is that it is extremely comfortable, accurate, and the patient feels that they get a more normal sleep since they are sleeping in their own bed. The cost is negligible, therefore patients can be given several economical and convenient sleep studies to ensure that the oral appliance is effective in eliminating snoring and OSA.

# Chapter Nine

## Where To Go for Support?

*Sleep Apnea is serious business now.* Take the next step and get yourself formally tested. You should be anxious to *rule out* sleep apnea as much as you should be motivated to get treatment if you are diagnosed with a sleep disorder. Here is a list of sources for more information, and they are also reference points for some of the material you have read already (among others).

- www.sleepapnea.org - American Sleep Apnea Association

- www.aasmnet.org - American Academy of Sleep Medicine

- www.sleepfoundation.org - National Sleep Foundation

- www.nhlbi.nih.gov/sleep - National Center on Sleep Disorders Research

- www.sleepeducation.com - Sleep Education from American Academy of Sleep Medicine

### *(NEW) Provent Sleep Apnea Therapy*

At the risk of excluding this new concept as a sleep apnea therapy option, I arbitrarily placed it at the end of the book. It is relatively new and not quite globally available just yet. I have just finished trying it on myself and the resulting data (more or less) proves that it is also an effective treatment for sleep apnea.

It must be prescribed by a physician and is now available outside of the USA. It's niche appears to be for those who have rejected or are non-compliant with CPAP. I wanted to evaluate it both in isolation and to use in concert with my oral device.

**Provent** is a disposable nasal device which is placed adhesively just inside each nostril. It allows you to *breathe in normally through your nose, but restricts expiration through the nose.* Instead it redirects the expiration airflow to increase your airway pressure in order to keep it open. In doing so, it effectively mimics the expiration phase of the CPAP in the respiratory cycle.

While this therapy is relatively new, it has been validated in multiple peer reviewed publications. Results show significantly reduced AHI and ODI-oxygen desaturation indexes, and reduced daytime sleepiness and snoring. It works across mild, moderate and severe OSA and is well tolerated by patients.

## Provent Therapy Works Across All OSA Severities[1]

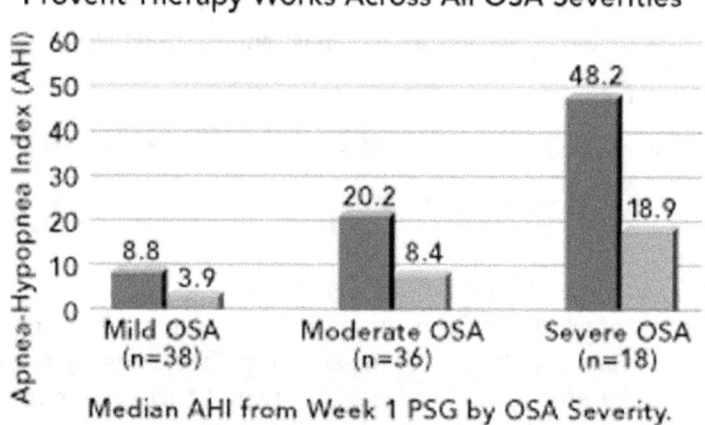

Median AHI from Week 1 PSG by OSA Severity.

■ Device Off　■ Nasal EPAP

## My Personal Test Results Using Provent Therapy

I ordered a starter pack consisting of 30 applications (a one month supply). The starter pack included Phase One (2 nasal applications offering low resistance, Phase Two (2 nasal applications at moderate resistance), and Phase Three at normal resistance for the balance of the month. The first and second phases were considered 'non-therapeutic' and were designed to get you accustomed to the concept. It was fairly easy to get accustomed to with one exception, I found if I woke up prior to my normal wakeup time that there was a significant cognitive factor whereby I was distracted just enough by the device sticking to my nose that my preoccupation prevented me from getting back to sleep. This happened during each of the first six nights, and in each situation I removed the nasal device and inserted my oral appliance to complete my sleep period.

Beyond that first week, I managed to sleep through the night and even though I woke up occasionally, I was able to get back to sleep without switching to my oral appliance. In fairness to the manufacturer, they address this eventuality and urge you to keep on with using the therapy until you get used to it.

At the end of the second week, I tested myself using the Embletta X100 home sleep device. The Embletta includes a nasal cannula to measure your breathing and oxygen saturation. I could not insert it because both nostrils are blocked by the Provent device, but I secured the nasal cannula outside of my nostrils with tape. I suspect the test data gave me a more favorable result in terms of hypopneic events, but I believe it's still reasonably accurate by virtue of the fact that I woke up feeling very rested. If you have an apnea and sleep without having your CPAP or MAD oral device, you seldom awaken feeling totally rested. This was not the case with my self-test.

To review, during my polysomnogram at the sleep lab I had 16 probes attached to my face and body while sleeping in an unfamiliar environment. I could not sleep on my side or stomach because it was too cumbersome, thus I scored a whopping 59 AHI (a severe apnea result).

When subsequently tested with my oral device in my own bed using the Embletta X100, I scored an very acceptable 6.5 AHI (remember at 5 AHI you are not considered to have sleep apnea). This time using the Provent Therapy I scored another very acceptable 8.9 AHI (mild sleep apnea is from 5 to 15 AHI). Even if there was a 10% negative error because of the aforementioned nasal cannula anomaly, it will still have taken my severe apnea reading down to a reasonably mild AHI reading.

In summation, I believe the manufacturer makes a legitimate claim that this new therapy works. I woke each time feeling refreshed and without the typical raw throat consistent with a heavy duty snoring machine. It does take some getting used to, but so does the CPAP. In terms of cost, depending on the quantities you purchase, the cost of shipping and the country you live in, the cost is roughly USD $2 to $3 per night. So the annual cost is going to be $750 to $1100. If you can get it covered by a health plan then it's a reasonable deal; if not then a top of the line customized oral device that lasts up to 10 years at a one-time cost of $2K to $3K is a better deal and virtually guaranteed effective when properly titrated.

Either way, I think we may finally have another legitimate OSA therapy beyond CPAP, MAD and Surgery that actually works. If you would like to research this on your own, I guarantee you will come to know more about this new sleep apnea therapy option than almost all clinicians will. I find the medical profession still incredibly naïve where it comes to sleep apnea, and particularly as it relates to effective therapies. Most have little idea that there are alternatives to CPAP with its incredibly high non-compliance rates.

Nevertheless, give this to your doctor so he can bring himself up to speed on the subject. Here are the research sources for this relatively new concept for treating sleep apnea that you can give him/her; or do the research for yourself.

- A Novel Nasal Expiratory Positive Airway Pressure (EPAP) Device for the Treatment of Obstructive Sleep Apnea: A Randomized Controlled TrialBerry, RB, Kryger, MH, Massie, CA [Sleep 2011;34 (4):479-485](19 Center, 3 Month, Randomized Controlled Trial)

- Long term use of a nasal expiratory positive airway pressure (EPAP) device as a treatment for obstructive sleep apnea Kryger MH, Berry RB, Massie CA. [SLEEP Abstract Supplement, 2011 (34):A118](13 Center, Long Term Efficacy Study)

- Nasal expiratory positive airway pressure (EPAP) for the treatment of obstructive sleep apnea: A review of clinical studies of Provent Therapy Doshi, R, Westbrook P [Respiratory Therapy Vol.6 No.4, 2011:6(4):45-49](Summary of All Peer Reviewed Studies)

- A Novel Nasal Expiratory Positive Airway Pressure (EPAP) Device for the Treatment of Obstructive Sleep Apnea: A Randomized Controlled Trial Berry, RB, Kryger, MH, Massie, CA [Sleep 2011;34 (4):479-485]

- Long term use of a nasal expiratory positive airway pressure (EPAP) device as a treatment for obstructive sleep apnea Kryger MH, Berry RB, Massie CA. [Journal of Clinical Sleep Medicine 2011; 7:5:449-453]

- Changes in lung volume and upper airway using MRI during application of nasal expiratory positive airway pressure in patients with sleep disordered breathing. Braga CW, Chen Q, Burschtin O, et al. [Journal of Applied Physiology 2011;111:1400-1409]

- Predictors of response to a nasal expiratory resistor device and its potential mechanisms of action for treatment of obstructive sleep apnea Patel AV, Hwang D, Masdeu MJ et al. [Journal of Clinical Sleep Medicine 2011;7(1):13-22]

- A convenient expiratory positive airway pressure nasal device for the treatment of sleep apnea in patients non-adherent with continuous positive airway pressureWalsh JK, Griffin KS, Forst EH, et al. [Sleep Medicine 2011;12:147-52]

- A multicenter, prospective study of a novel nasal EPAP device in the treatment of obstructive sleep apnea. Efficacy and 30-day adherence Rosenthal L, Massie CA, Dolan DC, et al. [Journal of Clinical Sleep Medicine 2009;5:532-37]

- A pilot evaluation of a nasal expiratory resistance device for the treatment of obstructive sleep apnea Colrain IM, Brooks S, Black J. [Journal of Clinical Sleep Medicine 2008;4(5):426-433]

- Nasal expiratory positive airway pressure (EPAP) for the treatment of obstructive sleep apnea: A review of clinical studies of Provent TherapyDoshi, R, Westbrook P [Respiratory Therapy Vol.6 No.4, 2011:6(4):45-49]

- Optimizing Patient Compliance on Nasal EPAP (Provent Therapy): The Role of the Healthcare ProviderDoshi, R, Heller D [Respiratory Therapy Vol.7 No.2, 2012:7(2):34-36]

- Nasal Expiratory Positive Airway Pressure (EPAP) Device to Treat Obstructive Sleep Apnea in Medicare Age Patients (age = 65)Glenn Adams, MD, FCCP, as presented at the SLEEP 2012 Annual Conference

- An Analysis of Responders to Nasal Expiratory Positive Airway Pressure (EPAP) During Long-term Follow-up Clifford Massie, PhD, as presented at the SLEEP 2012 Annual Conference

- Clinical Efficacy of a Nasal Expiratory Positive Airway Pressure (EPAP) Device for the Treatment of Obstructive Sleep Apnea (OSA)Massie C, Hart RW, as presented at the SLEEP 2011 Annual Conference

- Nasal EPAP as a Major OSA Therapeutic Option in a Clinical Sleep Center Setting Hwang D, Becker K, Chang J et al. as presented at the SLEEP 2011 Annual Conference.

- Retrospective Case Series Analysis of a Nasal Expiratory Positive Airway Pressure (EPAP) Device to Treat Obstructive Sleep Apnea in a Clinical Practice Adams, G, as presented at the SLEEP 2011 Annual Conference.

If you pay attention to even half of the information in this book, but take the appropriate action, you'll be able to *'Keep on Truckin'* like this guy and staying alive!

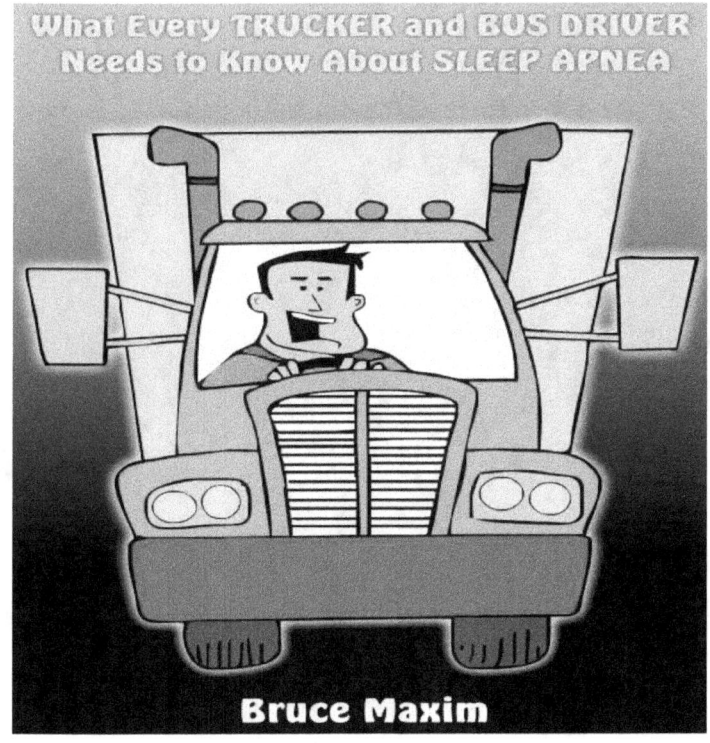